PUSWHISPERER III

PUSWHISPERER III:

A THIRD YEAR IN THE LIFE OF AN INFECTIOUS DISEASE DOCTOR

by Mark Crislip, MD

Bitingduck Press
Altadena, CA

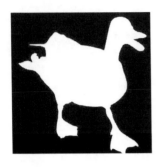

Published by Bitingduck Press
ISBN 978-1-938463-32-7
© 2018 Mark Crislip
All rights reserved
For information contact
Bitingduck Press, LLC
Altadena, CA
notifications@bitingduckpress.com
http://www.bitingduckpress.com
Cover image is an electron micrograph of the (non-pathogenic) marine psychrophile, *Colwellia psychrerythraea*

Disclaimer

The information here is not meant to diagnose, treat, cure or prevent any disease and is not intended for self-diagnosis or self-treatment of medical conditions that should be managed by a qualified health care provider.

To protect patient confidentiality, all demographic and identifying patient information was changed.

To my mother, Mary Jane Hall Crislip
for always laughing at my "jokes"

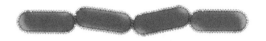

VZV

I consult at 4 hospitals—when my partner is gone it's 6—and on the weekend a whopping 8. So I get to see a lot of neat cases, being the sole common pathway for infectious diseases consultation. My title says I am Chief of Infectious Diseases, but it is easy to be King in a country with a population of 2.

Today's patient is a 78-year-old female who comes in with two days of increasingly severe abdominal pain. She has NHL (non-Hodgkin's lymphoma; probably better than National Hockey League) but has not been on chemotherapy for 8 months. She presents to the ER with pain requiring morphine and an ANC of 800 (absolute neutrophil count, not African National Congress; I have issues with initials. Where's my tissue?). CAT scan shows a slightly thickened colon and she is admitted with the question of typhlitis, a serious infection of the colon where the bowel bacteria invade into the bowel wall, killing it and often the patient.

The rest of her history is negative.

She receives antibiotics and stabilizes, but on day three develops a rash over her chest that over the next two days spreads everywhere, little dewdrop blisters with an erythematous base, and at the same time her abdominal pain resides.

I am called to comment on the duration of antibiotics and her rash.

When I see her I ask about the pain and she points to her right upper quadrant, far away from the alleged typhlitis, but innards are not all that smart and often do not know their true location, fooling their owner when they cause pain. Gallbladder pain, for example, can manifest in the shoulder. Angina in the left arm.

The rash? Sure looks like chickenpox. She did not have chickenpox as a child, but both her children did, so she has to have had the disease. No one escapes chickenpox if exposed.

I think her pain was zoster, then she developed disseminated zoster rather than the classic dermatomal rash of shingles. Typhlitis (or neutropenic enterocolitis) is usually seen in patients with prolonged, severe chemotherapy-induced neutropenia, which she did not have. It is also a problem in captive lowland gorillas, which she is not, but if you ever see Magilla holding his right lower quadrant in pain, be warned.

Disseminated zoster can occur with severe abdominal pain, although usually in transplant patients.

In all 4 cases, the initial symptom was severe abdominal pain which preceded the appearance of the classical herpetic vesicular skin lesions from two to four days in three cases, while one never developed skin lesions.

and the delay in skin lesions is not unheard of

The interval from the abdominal pain to the development of the skin lesions has ranged from one to 10 days, and this has led to a delay in the initiation of specific antiviral therapy in many cases...

I remember as an intern (being in medicine for 27 years gives one, if nothing else, lots of stories) an elderly male admitted with severe chest pain, and the diagnosis was dissection—tearing—of the aorta or worse, but work-up (in the era when the pixels on the CT were the size of the 'e's in the this sentence) was negative and on day 2 he erupted his shingles rash. And gas was $1.24 a gallon. And stay off my lawn.

She is surprisingly non-ill at this point, and doing well. I suggested acyclovir anyway. The real bummer was the delay in diagnosis, since the patient had a contagious infection and was not in isolation. Crap.

Rationalization

Curr Opin Gastroenterol. 2006 Jan;22(1):44-7. Neutropenic enterocolitis. http://www.ncbi.nlm.nih.gov/pubmed/16319675

Br J Dermatol. 2003 Oct; 149(4):862-5. Disseminated zoster, hyponatraemia, severe abdominal pain and leukaemia relapse: recognition of a new clinical quartet after bone marrow transplantation. http://www.ncbi.nlm.nih.gov/pubmed/14616382

Med Clin (Barc). 1998 Jun 13;111(1):19-22. [Abdominal pain as the initial symptom of visceral varicella zoster infection in hematopoietic stem cell transplant recipients]. http://www.ncbi.nlm.nih.gov/pubmed/9666431

Magilla Gorilla. https://en.wikipedia.org/wiki/Magilla_Gorilla

Do the Eyes Have It?

Two types of consults make me nervous. The first is a call from the Obstetrical service; I am discomforted at treating pregnant females and the fetus. Pregnant males do not bother me. The other is eye infections, in large part as I often do not get the diagnosis, just the suggestion of the diagnosis.

The patient is a young male from Africa. He has been asymptomatic until this year when he developed eye pain.

He sees the eye doctor who does the 4-star work up for nodular scleritis: no HIV or sarcoid or syphilis or Wegener's or inflammatory bowel disease or anything for that matter that is associated with scleritis except for a positive quantiFERON interferon-gamma release assay, suggesting tuberculosis. The chest x-ray is negative and he is sent to me with the diagnosis of nodular scleritis.

6 years ago he was treated for scrofula—TB of the neck lymph nodes—with, he says, 4 months of 4 pills then 2 months on injections. The pills, he tells me, were identical. So he received some sort of antibiotic therapy, just what is unknown and unknowable. Better than the old days when the King would lay his hands upon the scrofula to treat it.

Hmmm.

I go through the usual history and physical and come up with nothing new.

Ophthalmology assures me that the only treatable disease left in the differential diagnosis is TB and, no, they can't do a biopsy.

So is this TB? I do not know. I have asked those who know than me more about eye TB, and I got a verbal shrug of the shoulders and the advice to treat him for TB and see if he gets better.

TB of the eye is not that common, rare enough so that it is not mentioned in the TB section of the standard Infectious Diseases textbook. If you PubMed "TB" and "nodular sclerosis," there are 6 hits. One series of patients had TB as a cause in 8% of patients with scleritis, so it is an odd cause of an odd disease.

There is one case due to *Mycobacterium africanum*, a member of the *Mycobacterium tuberculosis* complex that causes about a quarter of TB cases in West Africa. So I suppose this could be *Mycobacterium africanum*, although I will never know and the treatment is the same.

Nine months later, after a course of 4 antibiotics, he was all better. Causal? I don't know, but I always take credit when patients get better.

TB or not TB. That is the question.

Rationalization

Clin Infect Dis. 1995 Sep; 21(3):653-5. Tuberculosis caused by Mycobacterium africanum associated with involvement of the upper and lower respiratory tract, skin, and mucosa.http://www.ncbi.nlm.nih.gov/pubmed/8527560

Scleritis http://emedicine.medscape.com/article/1228324-overview

Royal Touch. https://en.wikipedia.org/wiki/Royal_touch

My Motto: Frequently in Error, Never in Doubt

My Dad told me that there are four 'A's to being a consultant: availability, affability, appearance and ability. I added a fifth: accountability. Four out of five ain't bad. The other trick for being a consultant is pointing to left field, and hitting the ball out of the field. Most of the time you will be wrong, a swing and a miss, and no one will remember, but the rare times you connect, those are remembered.

The patient was a middle-aged diabetic who was in the hospital the first day of the month with pneumonia. He was never all that ill and sent home on a quinolone, worsened, and was readmitted.

At both the first admission and now, he had no pathogens seen on gram stain and cultures were negative. His CBC is unimpressive and while he is coughing up lots of sputum, he is not that toxic appearing.

He had two CT scans (don't ask)—one before and one now—that are most interesting. He has a growing round pneumonia in the right lower lobe, and now has two nodules in the upper lobe, along with increasing hilar adenopathy.

The history, as always, is key. Just prior to the onset of this disease he had driven the hot, dusty I-5 through the central valley of California. Twice.

I have seen two patients in my illustrious career who have had pneumonectomies for chronic pneumonia with large hilar lymph nodes and atypical cells on bronchoscopy who were thought to have lung cancer but, in fact, had coccidioidomycosis, aka Valley Fever. Both were truckers who traveled the I-5 to and from Los Angeles.

I bet he has acute coccidioidomycosis and have asked the lab to look for it on the cultures. It is also nice to warn the lab, as the form of coccidioidomycosis in human tissues is not communicable, but the form on the agar plate is, and one does not want the tech lab inadvertently acquiring cocci.

Even in places where the disease is common, coccidioidomycosis is often missed, so I cannot fault the treating physicians. Common things are, supposedly, common, hence the phrase. However, cases of coccidioidomycosis are increasing in Arizona and California, and a good reason to hold your breath when and if you visit those states.

...we conducted a prospective evaluation of 59 patients with CAP in the Phoenix, Arizona, area. Of 35 for whom paired coccidioidal serologic testing was performed, 6 (17%) had evidence of acute coccidioidomycosis. Coccidioidal pneumonia was more likely than noncoccidioidal CAP to produce rash. The following were not found to be risk factors or reliable predictors of infection: demographic features, underlying medical conditions, duration of time spent in disease-endemic areas, occupational and recreational activities, initial laboratory studies, and chest radiography findings. Coccidioidomycosis is a common cause of CAP in our patient population.

I put him on fluconazole, although coccidioidomycosis is often a self-limited disease, because he is a poorly controlled diabetic. Now I shall await the cultures and serology. As always, I hope reality doesn't get in the way of a great diagnosis.

It didn't. He eventually grew *Coccidioides immitis.*

It's good to be right now and then.

Rationalization

Emerg Infect Dis. 2009 Mar;15(3):397-401. Coccidioidal pneumonia, Phoenix, Arizona, USA, 2000-2004. http://www.springerlink.com/content/l4k0384717273w17/

Same Bug, Different Sites

I AM often unreasonably confident in my pronouncements. Diseases have patterns, and if you pay attention to the pattern, odds are in your favor that you will be right. Of course, you obtain cultures, and every now and then the patient's infection decides to pay you no mind, and grow something you don't expect. Words are best et with A1 sauce.

The first patient comes in with facial cellulitis, mostly on the cheek, that has not responded to oral antibiotics. He is mildly immuno-incompetent, but gives no reason by history for a soft tissue infection. On exam he has a swollen cheek with an obvious pocket of pus. A CT scan confirms a multi-loculated abscess. It should be staph—either methicillin resistant *S. aureus* (MRSA) or its methicillin-sensitive counterpart (MSSA). Typically Staphylococci make soft tissue abscesses. and given the lack of response to outpatient cephalexin I suspect MRSA. The gram stain shows gram positive cocci and I pontificate at length on the Panton-Valentine leukocidin, found in MRSA, which is an enzyme that liquefies human tissues and that is causing the abscess. Wrong.

The other patient, at another hospital, has the abrupt onset of a red, painful, swollen artificial knee 12 hours after an episode of a rigor and chills. He has no trauma and his joint is 6 months old.

The knee is washed out in the OR and has gram positive cocci in the pus and, like the first patient, I say, probably *Staphylococcus*, maybe *S. aureus*, maybe coagulase negative. The infection could have been acquired at the time of surgery, but the onset is a bit late for coagulase negative Staphylococci.

Both cultures grow *Streptococcus agalactiae,* aka Group B streptococcus.

The heck. I see this bug now and then, but growing it in the non-pregnant adult is always a surprise. It classically causes infection after delivery. Of a baby. The UPS driver need not worry.

As a cause of cellulitis/abscess in the adult, Group B streptococcus is distinctly odd. While reported in infants and young children, you can cut off my hand and still count the number of cases I could find on PubMed. In one series of Group B streptococcal infections, soft tissue infections are uncommon:

Thirteen of these 19 (68.4%) patients had clinical evidence of urinary tract infection (UTI). Streptococcus agalactiae infections were diagnosed in 26 of 34 inpatients. Besides the 13 inpatients with an UTI, 2 had bacteremia of unknown origin, 2 pneumonia, 2 erysipelas, 1 spondylodiscitis, 1 peritonitis, 2 prostatitis, 1 perirectal abscess, 1 testicular abscess, and 1 diabetic foot infection.

Soft tissue abscesses are rarer still.

Any organism can end up in a prosthetic joint, but Group B streptococcus is not one of the common causes either. Over a 12 year period in France, one hospital found 30 cases, all hematogenous in origin, and I suspect that his rigor was a transient bacteremia from an unknown source. 19 of the 30 joint infections were cured with antibiotics alone.

One would think a streptococcus would be a piece of cake to kill off, but the two series suggest that this organism is associated with about a 30% failure rate, perhaps due to underlying comorbidities in these patients.

There is some data to suggest that pregnant females with Ig subtype deficiencies are more prone to Group B streptococcal bacteremia. While low antibody levels are not reported for non-pregnant adults, I look for antibody issues in the elderly with invasive Group B streptococcal infections by doing a serum protein electrophoresis to measure immunoglobulin levels. I have found the odd myeloma over the years as a result.

Rationalization

Joint Bone Spine. 2009 Oct; 76(5):491-6. doi: 10.1016/j.jbspin.2008.11.010. Epub 2009 Jun 13. Outcome of group B strepto-coccal prosthetic hip infections compared to that of other bacterial infections. http://www.ncbi.nlm.nih.gov/pubmed/19525137

Presse Med. 2009 Nov; 38(11):1577-84. doi: 10.1016/j. lpm.2009.02.026. Epub 2009 Jun 13. Group B streptococcal prosthet-ic joint infections: a retrospective study of 30 cases. http://www.ncbi. nlm.nih.gov/pubmed/19525087

Int Arch Allergy Appl Immunol. 1983;72(3):249-52. Deficiency of IgG subclasses in mothers of infants with group B streptococcal septi-cemia. http://www.ncbi.nlm.nih.gov/pubmed/6352515

POLL RESULTS

I…

• rarely call the diagnosis before the tests are back as I don't want to be wrong. 12%

• always try and call the diagnosis before the tests are back. Who cares if I am wrong. 42%

• derive great comfort from long differentials as one of the diseases on the list is bound to be right. 12%

• have never been surprised by a diagnosis. I am that good. 4%

• always get the diagnosis right at the beginning. It is the tests that are wrong. 23%

• Other Answers 8%

They don't even have tests for what I always diagnose, low ni-tric oxide

Sometimes What Looks To Be Unimportant Isn't

L AST January I took care of a diabetic patient with *S. au-reus* bacteremia and discitis as a complication of dialysis. He did fine with a long course of antibiotics, and as best I can tell, he is a cure. In January he had, on the chest x-ray obtained for his central catheter placement, a small opacity—not even really an infiltrate—in the right middle lobe of the lung. It looked like scar or atelectasis but it did not look like anything important. He also had no pulmonary symptoms.

So I passed the lung lesion off as nothing. Cue theme from *Jaws*.

Fast forward 8 months to end of August. While he still has no pulmonary symptoms, he has another chest x-ray for dialysis catheter placement and now has a large (7 cm) mass in the right middle lobe, abutting the pleura and with a smooth edge. A CT scan shows a mass with a necrotic center, and given the prior smoking history, cancer is highest on the list. Of course, this is an ID blog so you can anticipate that cancer isn't the answer. He goes to CT guided biopsy and the biopsy shows what looks to be cryptococcus.

Cultures were not done, and eventually we grow nothing from blood or sputum. His serum cryptococcal antigen is 1:16, so I know he has cryptococcus, and, fortunately, the spinal fluid cryptococcal antigen is negative. No meningitis, the feared complication of this yeast.

I think he has had 9 months of slowly growing cryptococcal pneumonia. The CT findings are typical of this unusual disease.

The nodules and masses have a predominantly peripheral distribution in 80% of the cases. Cavitation of nodules or consolidation is seen in approximately 40% of the cases.

Should be treated? Oh yeah. Although cryptococcal pneumonia can be self-limited in normal hosts, this is a diabetic dialysis patient, with progressive pneumonia and positive antigen suggesting this is more than an isolated pulmonary infection, even given the lack of symptoms. No way will it clear on its own. So he will get a long course of the anti-fungal fluconazole.

And he was cured.

Rationalization

Pulmonary Cryptococcosis in Immunocompetent Patients: CT Findings in 12 Patients Danial L. Fox and Nestor L. Müller1 http://www.ajronline.org/cgi/content/abstract/185/3/622

Look At It Yourself

I DO not know how many of my readers are young whipper-snappers in training. I am occasionally curious about the demographics of my readers. The only thing I know with certainty is that you are a human of rare taste and intelligence. And no, that doesn't make you look fat at all. I can pander with the best of them.

But, as a crotchety old fart, I occasionally feel the overpowering urge to give advice, couched in stories, so that you do not make the mistakes of others. Not that you will learn from my mistakes (I don't make mistakes); people must make, and learn from, their own errors. But what the heck.

So I get called late in the evening with a question. There is a patient being admitted with a thigh abscess and shortness of breath. A year ago he received a course of the antibiotic isoniazid (INH) for a positive tuberculosis test, but is otherwise healthy.

As part of the evaluation of the shortness of breath, he had a chest x-ray that showed an upper lobe infiltrate which lead to a CT scan. The CT reports cavitary upper lobe infiltrates that "support the diagnosis of TB or fungal infection." Support. Like it is some worthless supplement. Since we do not have fungi worth speaking about in the northwest, given the history TB must be the diagnosis. I was asked what to do next.

Isolate the patient and get some sputum to look for TB. Since he is clinically stable, there is no need to give TB therapy tonight. I rolled over and went back to sleep.

I have a vague memory of a poster at a meeting years ago where an ID doc listened to the curbside consult, gave advice and then—because he evidently did not have enough to do—went and did the full-meal-deal history and physical. He found that just based on the information from the curbside he gave the wrong advice something like half the time. I keep this in mind when I hear about complicated cases. Next morning, I run into the caller and ask about the case and we pull up the CT scan results.

The CT may have been many things, but it was most certainly not TB. The radiologist had read the film with the information that it was a potential case of TB. This may come as a surprise to some, but the history can really guide the interpretation of the x-ray.

Here is the rule. Any film that is not a normal chest x-ray should be reviewed with the radiologist. Never, ever, rely on the report alone. One day, if you do, it will come back to bite you in the butt. You will learn a lot and get to the diagnosis much faster if you speak with the radiologist. Over the years I have seen many cases that went down the wrong diagnostic road because the treating physicians relied on an erroneous read of the film because the radiologist was given the wrong information and the attending never looked at the damn film themselves. And get off my lawn.

In this case there were numerous cannonball peripheral cavitary lesions that were septic pulmonary emboli due to the MRSA in the thigh, the blood, and the sputum. Clinically he had acute onset of fevers and shortness of breath a few days after the thigh abscess formed. Although the echocardiogram was negative, clinically he had right-sided endocarditis as a complication of the abscess and was treated accordingly.

Everyone was blindsided by the history of treated latent TB and an upper lobe infiltrate, which happens, but if the docs had been able to review the CT with the radiologist (and, in their defense, it was late in the evening, the joys and dangers of telemedicine), I bet the diagnosis of TB would have been rapidly thrown out.

That's the old fart's advice: always take the time to go over the films with the radiologist. Unless you practice where the radiologists act like jerks when they have to review the films with you. Those kinds of radiologists are few and far between where I practice. I know them and avoid them.

POLL RESULTS

I only
- Look at all X rays. 35%
- Look at all abnormal X rays. 8%
- Read all reports. 17%
- Read the conclusion of the report. 2%
- Use X-Ray glasses I ordered from a comic. 32%
- Other Answers 6%
  1. I read this 'cause I like your style!
  2. its hit or miss. I overread consistently.
  3. look all x-rays and all reports
  4. Read all notes

Worms

WORMS are usually a disappointment. Most patients do not really have worms when they show up in clinic. Perhaps they have misidentified material that looks worm-like but is not a worm. Mucus strings (ew) are on the top of that list. Or they are worried that they might have acquired a worm from travel to the developing world like the Southern US. Or they have delusions of parasitism. True worms are unusual. Once an earthworm fell out of a patient's pocket after gardening and he thought he had passed it. You would think a gardener would know an earthworm.

The patient this week is an exception. She said that she passed a worm. A long worm. It took three tugs to pull out a six-foot-long worm that was then lost to the automatic flush mechanism of the toilet. The patient thinks it was a tapeworm, and compared her memory to photos on the Googles. I have no reason to disbelieve her. A middle-class American, she had traveled the world over the years and had visited many countries where tapeworms are common.

An ova and parasite (O&P) stool exam is negative, so the

worm has probably passed. But I treated her anyway and will recheck an O&P in 3 months.

There are 4 tapeworms that can infect humans: the pork tapeworm (*T. solium*), the beef tapeworm (*T. saginata*), the fish tapeworm (*Diphyllobothrium* spp.), and the dwarf tapeworm (*Hymenolepis* spp.) (no, it does not infect dwarves. Gimli is safe). I do not know which worm she had. Beef tapeworms can grow to 40 feet and others can grow to 100 feet, and just typing this gives me the heebie jeebies.

The patient said she was always careful when traveling and tried not to eat dangerous foods.

Cautious eating may help, but I would not be so sanguine. Bottled water is often a bottle filled at the tap, and the literature is filled with the results of screening the stool of food handlers all over the world.

This study reports on the occurrence of enteroparasites based on data from an ethnographic study of food handlers in the city of Cascavel, Paraná, Brazil. Fecal material from 343 food handlers of both sexes, between 14 and 75 years of age, was analyzed using Lutz, modified Ritchie and Ziehl-Neelsen techniques. Ethnographic relationships were investigated by means of specific questionnaires. Positive fecal samples were found for 131 (38.2%) handlers.

That is one representative example of many similar studies. And stool, human and animal, is a universal fertilizer. I always emphasize that everything we eat has a patina of human and animal stool. Sometimes it is thick, sometime it is thin, but it is always there.

It is why I only eat deep fried food.

Rationalization

Rev Inst Med Trop Sao Paulo. 2009 Jan-Feb;51(1):31-5. Enteroparasitosis and their ethnographic relationship to food handlers in a tourist and economic center in Paraná, Southern Brazil. http://www.ncbi.nlm.nih.gov/pubmed/19229388

Ribs Are Back

Any organism can infect any organ in any person at any time. Thank goodness, as it gives me a career. Still, there are patterns. Certain organisms have a propensity for some organs over others.

The patient is a young IV drug user who presents first with back pain, then with chest pain. The back pain has been present for about six weeks, and is right over his scapula.

The chest pain, there for a week, is centered over is anterior chest just below the clavicle.

He denies fevers or chills.

The rest of his history and physical is negative. While tender to touch with slight swelling over the chest, it is not red or hot, and there is nothing on the back.

His complete blood count, liver panel, and blood cultures are negative; an MRI of his chest reveals a small nodule in the periphery of the right lung.

Not a surprise given that he uses black tar heroin, a complex gamish of narcotic and insoluble organic material. It is probably goo that lodged in the lung, and will have to be watched.

The head of the first rib is all moth-eaten, and looks like osteomyelitis—bone infection. Similarly, in the middle of the third rib on the back is another inflamed lesion. He denies any trauma to account for the findings.

The thoracic surgeon tells me that taking out a first rib is tricky; there are these pesky vascular structures like arteries and veins just under it. Just like a surgeon to worry about bleeding. So we sent him off for a bone biopsy and it grew *S. aureus*.

I have never seen a case of hematogenous rib osteomyelitis, and clinically it behaved more like a pair of what is called "Brodie abscesses": indolent infection of long bone without the usual rubor, dolor, calor and tumor of bone infection.

Most of the reported cases of rib infections are in kids, due to trauma, and are due to weird organisms.

Hematogenous, due to *Staphylococcus*, to the rib, in the adult (game of Clue anyone?) is the exception.

A total of 106 cases of rib osteomyelitis were reviewed, including 2 cases described in detail. Mycobacterial and bacterial infections accounted for 47 cases each. Fungal rib osteomyelitis occurred in 11 cases and 1 case was caused by Entamoeba histolytica. Most cases occurred in children and young adults. The mean duration of symptoms before diagnosis was 16, 26 and 32 weeks for bacterial, mycobacterial and fungal rib osteomyelitis, respectively. Common clinical signs were fever (73%), soft tissue mass (64%) and chest pain (60%). Route of infection was defined in 85 cases: 62% from contiguous spread and 38% via hematogenous route of infection. Eighty-nine percent had a favorable outcome after antimicrobial therapy with or without surgery. In conclusion, rib osteomyelitis is a rare infection of various aetiologies. The majority of cases occur in children and young adults and its diagnosis is usually delayed for several weeks.

So I guess he is typical for an atypical presentation of an atypical disease. Typical of my practice.

As is so often the case, the siren call of heroin was stronger than the need for medical care and he left in the middle of the night. I never saw him again.

Rationalization

Scand J Infect Dis. 2000;32(3):223-7. Osteomyelitis of the ribs in the antibiotic era. http://www.ncbi.nlm.nih.gov/pubmed/10879590

A review from 1938, if, like me, you enjoy that sort of thing: brodie's abscess and its differential diagnosis. http://www.ncbi.nlm.nih.gov/pmc/articles/PMC2210084/pdf/brmedj04206-0014.pdf

No Go

THE patient is an elderly male with three months of a nagging (pick up after yourself, leave the toilet seat down) cough and failure to thrive. He denies fevers, chills, sweats or other complaints.

His past medical history is significant for a B-cell non-Hodgkin's lymphoma, immunoglobulin deficiency and a left lower lobe pneumonia a year ago. The routine labs are mostly normal, he runs on the low side with his white count.

A CT scan of the lungs shows a variety of peripheral nodules. Nodules on CT mean fungus or mycobacteria in my world, less interestingly cancer. So off to bronchoscopy, and the sputum specimen shows branching gram positive rods. That's two potential organisms: *Nocardia* and *Actinomycosis*.

Actinomycosis is usually due to aspiration, and aspiration does not lead to peripheral nodules. *Nocardia* is usually due to inhalation and that leads to peripheral nodules (as does hematogenous spread).

And indeed it grows *Nocardia*, *N. nova* to be precise. There are over 25 different *Nocardia*, not including an oddly named Italian rock album. Anyone knows Italian, let me know what the deal is with that album.

Nocardia has a propensity to cause brain abscesses, which he does not have.

N. nova is one of the more uncommon species to cause human and animal disease; there are 95 citations in PubMed. In cats the disease is often cutaneous and

interestingly, the majority of infections were attributable to N. nova.

What was going on in the cats?

Immediate and/or predisposing causes could be identified in all cases, and included: renal transplantation [one cat]; chronic corticosteroid administration [three cats]; catabolic state following chylothorax surgery [one cat]; fight injuries [seven cats]; FIV infections [three of seven cats tested].

They give cats kidney transplants in Eastern Australia !?! They wasted a perfectly good human kidney on a cat ?!? Have they no shame?

Although trimethoprim/sulfamethoxazole is the treatment for *Nocardia*, susceptibility can be variable and should be checked; he is on trimethoprim/sulfamethoxazole while we wait.

Eventually he was a cure.

Rationalization

Clinical and microbiological features of nocardiosis 1997–2003

http://jmm.sgmjournals.org/cgi/content/full/56/4/545

Aust Vet J. 2006 Jul;84(7):235-45. Nocardia infections in cats: a retrospective multi-institutional study of 17 cases. http://www.ncbi.nlm.nih.gov/pubmed/16879126

....

Which Came First?

B ACK from the Grand Tour of the NE looking at colleges with my eldest. Youth is wasted on the young, as is college. After touring the campuses I told my son, the heck with him, I am quitting work and going back to school. He can support me. Back to the routine, but not the grind. ID remains much too fun and interesting to really want to go back to college, but still... he gazes wistfully into the middle distance, dreaming of college libraries.

Where was I? Oh. Yeah. Infections.

Deep venous thrombosis (DVT) is a common complication of bedrest or infection. Infection leads to inflammation which is proinflammatory with leads to clot in all the wrong places: coronary arteries, pulmonary arteries, and cerebral arteries.

That is the usual order of business.

The patient today? Kind of backwards. He has a thrombosis, first of the superior mesenteric artery, and has it bypassed. He goes home and returns with a red, swollen leg and he develops clot in the deep veins of his leg with a pulmonary embolism.

Then, a couple of days later, he has a fever and for the next few days has positive blood cultures with *S. aureus*. A sustained bacteremia means an endovascular infection, and, after evaluation of all the likely suspects, we are left with his DVT probably being secondarily infected.

Kind of odd. Septic thrombophlebitis of the great vessels is occasionally seen, but usually the infection occurs simultaneously with the clot. *S. aureus* is quite the clot former; in case you ever wondered why it is also called coagulase positive Staphylococcus. I suspect you never wondered.

As best I can determine, there are no reported cases of secondarily infected DVT's of the leg, so maybe this is not the diagnosis, although we can't find another reason for the sustained bacteremia. Equally rare are reported cases of either femoral or saphenous vein septic thrombophlebitis. Most of the cases are of the great veins of the neck and chest as a complication of intravenous catheters.

With anticoagulation and antibiotics (I am so negative, anti-this and anti-that, can't I ever see the positive side of cases?) he is much improved and will continue the antibiotics at least 6 weeks.

Rationalization

Risk of deep vein thrombosis and pulmonary embolism after acute infection in a community setting. http://www.thelancet.com/journals/lancet/article/PIIS0140-6736(06)68474-2/abstract

Scand J Infect Dis. 1980;12(2):123-7. Postoperative deep venous thrombosis and infectious complications. A clinical study of patients undergoing colo-rectal surgery. http://www.ncbi.nlm.nih.gov/pubmed/7375824

Medicine (Baltimore). 1985 Nov;64(6):394-400. Central venous sep-

tic thrombophlebitis—the role of medical therapy. http://www.ncbi.
nlm.nih.gov/pubmed/3932817

POLL RESULTS

Which came first

- chicken 9%
- egg 7%
- both simultaneously 3%
- the proto-chicken came first, giving the egg, then the
chicken. 34%
- to get to the other side. 34%
- Other Answers 2%
  Jenny McCarthy! Oh, wait. That was the Dodo. Never
  mind!

....

0 to 60

WHEN I awoke this morning I had one of that rare conflu-
ence of events where I had no patients to see. None. Lots
of discharges and no new consults, and I took my time getting
ready for work, figuring that I would cruise through the day and
maybe get home early and stack the 2 cords of wood that were
delivered this week.

Then, in 10 minutes, boom, five consults. Zero to sixty. Life
is good and I have something to write about this week. I'll leave
the wood for the kids this weekend. Yeah. Like that is going to
happen.

Older male with 6 weeks of fevers, rigors, sweats, and malaise.

Nothing else on review of systems and his exam is benign except for a 3/6 blowing murmur in the aortic position, courtesy of
a bovine prosthetic valve from a year ago.

He tells me that he took antibiotics with dental work on or
about the time he had the onset of his symptoms.

Past medical history: mild Crohn's (did I put the 'h' in the right
place?), currently on no therapy.

His doc gets some blood cultures as an outpatient and they all grow *S. anginosus*.

As streptococci go, *S. anginosus* is not a common cause of endocarditis.

In 101 (54.3%) cases S. anginosus alone caused infection and in 85 (45.7%) cases it was associated with other microorganisms. Abscesses accounted for 110 (59.1%) infections. Sites of infection were: miscellaneous skin and soft tissue, 64 (34.4%), intraabdominal 41 (22%), head and neck 34 (18.3%), pleuropulmonary 22 (11.8%), genitourinary 9 (4.8%), musculoskeletal 6 (3.2%), endocarditis 5 (2.7%) and primary bacteremia 5 (2.7%).

S. anginosus is one the streptococci that likes to cause abscesses. So even though the exam and history do not suggest an abscess anywhere, we are going to get an echocardiogram to make sure these is no abscess around the prosthetic valve, given both the organism and the prolonged symptoms.

Where did the wee beastie come from? It is tempting to blame the dental procedure, but it was a filling that didn't even require anesthesia and, while he took ampicillin, it is not as if prophylactic antibiotics do much:

the risks of developing IE were estimated to be 1 in 46,000 for unprotected procedures (1 in 10,700 and 1 in 54,300 for subjects with prosthetic and native valve PCC, respectively) and 1 in 150,000 for protected procedures.

The data for antibiotic prophylaxis for dental work is unimpressive even for the ever compulsive Cochrane reviewers:

There remains no evidence about whether penicillin prophylaxis is effective or ineffective against bacterial endocarditis in people at risk who are about to undergo an invasive dental procedure. There is a lack of evidence to support previously published guidelines in this area. It is not clear whether the potential harms and costs of antibiotic administration outweigh any beneficial effect.

So the data, such as it is, doesn't support antibiotics prophylaxis. I bet that the occasional dental procedure very rarely leads to endocarditis, but so does routine flossing and brushing, which is why I do neither. Still, prophylaxis is the standard of care, so I would not advise against it.

I bet the infection is more likely a complication of his Chrhohnhsh disease.

Among 213 consecutive patients treated for proven native valve endocarditis, six (2.8%) had inflammatory bowel diseases (three with ulcerative colitis and three with Crohn›s disease). Three patients with inflammatory bowel disease were from the retrospective group, and three were from the prospective group. The prevalence of inflammatory bowel diseases has been determined to be 0.0641% in the Düsseldorf area... On the basis of these data, a 44-fold overrepresentation of inflammatory bowel diseases among the 213 patients with endocarditis was calculated with a statistical significance of p much less than 0.001.

Oddly, having open ulcerated mucosa bathed in stool increases risk for bacteremia and endocarditis. Who would have thunk it?

As long as there is no abscess, I have a reasonable chance of curing his endocarditis.

The echocardiogram was negative and he received a course of IV antibiotics that cured the infection.

Rationalization

N Z Med J. 1988 Dec 14;101(859):813-6. Clinically significant Streptococcus anginosus (Streptococcus milleri) infections: a review of 186 cases. http://www.ncbi.nlm.nih.gov/pubmed/3060769

Clin Infect Dis. 2006 Jun 15;42(12):e102-7. Epub 2006 May 10. Estimated risk of endocarditis in adults with predisposing cardiac conditions undergoing dental procedures with or without antibiotic prophylaxis. http://www.ncbi.nlm.nih.gov/pubmed/16705565

Cochrane Database Syst Rev. 2008 Oct 8;(4):CD003813. doi: 10.1002/14651858.CD003813.pub3. Antibiotics for the prophylaxis of bacterial endocarditis in dentistry. http://www.ncbi.nlm.nih.gov/pubmed/18843649

Am J Med. 1992 Apr; 92(4):391-5. Increased risk of bacterial endocarditis in inflammatory bowel disease. http://www.ncbi.nlm.nih.gov/pubmed/1307218

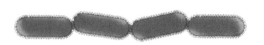

An Unexpected Belly Laugh

B USY day. My partner is learnin' at the Infections Diseases Society of America conference, so I am in Orygun holding down the fort. Lots of cool cases to write about in the days ahead. When I have to cover both practices I have to work at warp factor 9 to get all the patients seen in a reasonable amount of time. It takes concentration and I pay a little less to my social environment. Not a day for hoots and giggles.

I was going through my faxes when I read one that resulted in an unexpected belly laugh.

I am, it appears, an award winner. A 2010 Champion of Medicine—and Newt Gingrich himself will give me the award himself on Election Night if I can make it to Washington.

Funny thing is, several other docs in the office received identical offers, down to the 'handwritten message' that is so obviously a font.

So Newt must think we docs are a bunch of gullible rubes who just fell off the turnip truck. And maybe we are.

A quick Google and you discover this is fax-spam.

You can find the template on the Huffington Post. I never thought I would recommend the HuffPo with their lamentable track record on alternative medicine. But there you go. The enemy of my enemy, I suppose.

And it will cost me $5000 to attend.

Telling someone they're being chosen "Physician of the Year" or a "Champion of Medicine" is evidently a popular way to separate a fool from their money.

I expect I will next be asked by Newt to help move some oil money out of Nigeria.

I wonder if there are any docs out there with the combination of ego and gullibility who will fall for this? Or who do not see this as insulting? Probably.

Rationalization

Newt Gingrich Spams Doctors: Give Me $5000 And I'll Give You A 'Prestigious' Award. http://www.huffingtonpost.com/2010/10/12/gingrich-faxes-doctors-in_n_759871.html

Gingrich scam continues, even as presidential rumors float. http://www.dailykos.com/storyonly/2010/10/19/910100/-Gingrich-scam-continues,-even-as-presidential-rumors-float

Don't Just Do Something, Stand There

Finally I am back in action. Hard drive crash. Hard drive replaced, backups transferred, what a royal pain.

When I was a fellow I was up all night writing the final draft of a grant and accidentally pulled the plug. Word Not So Perfect did not have auto-back up and I lost all the work. I wanted to cry. As a result I always have three or four copies of everything, but getting the system back to normal is still a pain.

Fever. It is the most common reason why I get a consult. Why the fever? Why not? is not considered a good answer.

The patient is a young female with 5 days of fever, malaise with a sudden onset of left sided pain radiating over to the epigastric area.

She is admitted and I am called after 48 hours when the evaluation fails to yield a source of the fever. The worry is that she has endocarditis because the CT, done for the pain, shows a big splenic infarct. About half of her spleen is gone.

Her history is typical for my practice: heroin use, bipolar, smoker, sickle cell trait.

Exam has a 2/6 heart murmur but nothing else to suggest endocarditis.

Her complete blood count, liver tests, urinalysis (Am I the only one who heard Kirk say "Urinalysis, Mr. Spock?"), and blood cultures are normal or negative, depending on the study.

She remains febrile and has no risk factors for unusual diseases.

So I say do nothing. I bet, given her age, she has a viral syndrome and the stress led to splenic infraction—which I learned is not uncommon in sickle cell trait, thanks as always to the PubMed. It is amazing how, after 25 years in the biz, that I usually learn something new every day. I guess I am slow on the uptake.

Since under stress sickle cell trait patients can infarct their spleens, I presume the fever and slight dehydration was enough to do that. Most of the literature suggests splenic infarction is due to high altitude, like climbing Mt. Fuji, so not typical in that respect, although she was on the 4th floor of the hospital.

Sickle cell trait occurs in approximately 300 million people worldwide, with the highest prevalence of approximately 30% to 40% in sub-Saharan Africa. Long considered a benign carrier state with relative protection against severe malaria, sickle cell trait occasionally can be associated with significant morbidity and mortality. Sickle cell trait is exclusively associated with rare but often fatal renal medullary cancer. Current cumulative evidence is convincing for associations with hematuria, renal papillary necrosis, hyposthenuria, splenic infarction, exertional rhabdomyolysis, and exercise-related sudden death. Sickle cell trait is probably associated with complicated hyphema, venous thromboembolic events, fetal loss, neonatal deaths, and preeclampsia, and possibly associated with acute chest syndrome, asymptomatic bacteriuria, and anemia in pregnancy. There is insufficient evidence to suggest an independent association with retinopathy, cholelithiasis, priapism, leg ulcers, liver necrosis, avascular necrosis of the femoral head, and stroke.

So we waited and gave no antibiotics, and in a day or two the fevers were gone. I wonder if, given the size of the infarct, it that helped perpetuate the fever. Dead tissue can be a cause of fever as well.

When you are early in medical practice, the urge is to do something—anything—and modern medicine is not conducive to a leisurely assessment of the hospitalized patient. But sometimes it is important to not just do something, but stand there.

Rationalization

Am J Med. 2009 Jun; 122(6):507-12. doi: 10.1016/j.am-jmed.2008.12.020. Epub 2009 Apr 24. Complications associated with sickle cell trait: a brief narrative review. http://www.ncbi.nlm.nih.gov/pubmed/19393983

....

Not Everything Is Infectious

NOT every patient I see has an infection as the cause of their symptoms. My old boss used to say that, since infections affect any organ system, the ID doc has to be the second best subspecialist in the hospital. Second best cardiologist, second best pulmonologist, etc. So I try and keep an eye out for a diagnosis that is not that interesting...er, I mean, not infectious.

I am called to see a patient who is septic without a source. He has widely metastatic cancer and chemotherapy has resulted in severe mucositis (inflammation of all mucous membranes, including the mouth and throat). He cannot swallow and so he needs intravenous fluids. He is leaving the infusion clinic when he collapses. Rapid response is called and he is transferred to the ICU, hypotensive and hypothermic.

He gets the usual work up for sepsis, but all the cultures are negative, as are the X rays, and after 48 hours they call me.

The exam is negative except for severe mucositis and hypotension being treated with vasopressors. He looks ill, but not the usual septic or cancer ill. He looked like he had zombie make-up on, an odd pallor that was kind of a white/yellow/brown mix. Hard to describe, but he looked sick in a different way than the usual ICU patient I see.

It makes its approach in so slow and insidious a manner, that the patient can hardly fix a date to his earliest feeling of that languor, which is shortly to become so extreme. The countenance gets pale, the whites of the eyes become pearly, the general frame flabby rather than wasted; the pulse perhaps large, but remarkably soft and compressible, and occasionally with a slight jerk, especially under the slightest excitement; there is an increasing indisposition to exertion, with an uncomfortable feeling of faintness or breathlessness on attempting it; the heart is readily made to palpitate; the whole surface of the body presents a blanched, smooth and waxy appearance; the lips, gums and tongue seem bloodless; the flabbiness of the solids increases; the appetite fails; extreme languor and faintness supervene, breathlessness and palpitations being produced by the most trifling exertion or emotion; some slight œdema is probably perceived about the ankles; the debility becomes extreme, the patient can no longer rise from his bed, the mind occasionally wanders, he falls into a prostrate and half-torpid state.

Could not have said it better myself.

Labs show a white cell count of 3,000 with a marked left shift, presumably from the recent chemotherapy.

Slightly low sodium, 138, the rest of the electrolytes are normal.

Interestingly, the serum glucose at the time of the collapse was 25 and the patient was not on insulin nor in liver failure.

It is 4 o'clock in the afternoon and I call the hospitalist and say, he may be septic, but I bet it is adrenal insufficiency.

There is a problem with being an internist sometimes: you like to do all the diagnostics to prove the diagnosis before embarking on therapy, So we did the cosyntropin stimulation test, but waited for the results.

Maybe not such a good idea, for in the morning the patient was much worser and the cortisol came back at 0.4 before and after the cosyntropin. Probably he has metastasis to the adrenals.

With a slug of cortisol the patient perked up, but in retrospect the low glucose should have been a hint that I should have checked a cortisol and then given a dose of steroids immediately.

Years ago, in the depths of the AIDS epidemic, I saw a patient who had spent the prior two months in Brigham and Women's in Boston with refractory failure to thrive and no etiology found.

He came home to Portland to die and was transferred to my hospital. When I walked in the room he had a tan that looked like he had just returned from two months in Hawaii, not Boston. He too had severe adrenal insufficiency that had been missed, probably for months. With steroids he survived another 6 months.

Primary adrenal insufficiency (Addison's disease) can be tricky to diagnose, especially when it is acute or indolent in presentation and medical interventions (IV fluids) prevent the classic manifestations of low sodium and high potassium, as was the case in both these patients.

I used to see adrenal insufficiency in HIV reasonably often in the bad old days. No longer, but I still keep half an ear out for the disease. And sometimes it is better to treat immediately than to wait for the tests to come back.

Rationalization

Curr Opin Endocrinol Diabetes Obes. 2010 Jun;17(3):205-9. doi: 10.1097/MED.0b013e3283394441. Adrenal function in HIV infection. http://www.ncbi.nlm.nih.gov/pubmed/20404726

Read the original by Addison, 1855: ON THE CONSTITUTIONAL AND LOCAL EFFECTS OF DISEASE OF THE SUPRA-RENAL CAPSULES.

....

Not What I Had Hoped For

THE patient is an elderly male with the worst headache of his life. I once had a patient who was hit on the head with a German sausage; he had the wurst headache of his life. Thank you, I will be here all week.

It had been present for five days when he came to the ER and had a spinal tap. 950 white blood cells per milliliter (low), normal glucose, protein of 100 (high). Consistent with aseptic meningitis. But from what?

Of interest is that two other adults in the household also have the worst headache of their lives. It is the end of October and they have had no unusual exposures to water or pools. The classic outbreak in families for aseptic meningitis is due to enteroviruses. I once took care of a family where three of four people had enteroviral infections after swimming in a pool together in August, and two of the patients were kids.

He is the wrong age and it is almost the wrong time of year for enterovirus. I will say as an aside that the other two in the household never had a spinal tap, so I presume they were all infected with the same organism.

However, they live in the country and have been plagued with mice this year, capturing at least one a day. Why all the mice? Not certain. It was an odd summer in the NW, with no real summer and few ripened tomatoes. They live near the railroad and told me that the mice flock to the area because of the grain that comes off the freight cars. With a change in the weather the mice moved indoors.

So I am thinking LCVM, lymphocytic choriomeningitis virus, a mouse-associated infection that is probably underreported as a cause of aseptic meningitis.

"The prevalence of LCMV in wild mice in the United States ranges between 3.9% and 13.4%. Human cases demonstrate a fall-to-winter predominance corresponding to the movement of rodents indoors. Limited data are available on human infections but serologic studies in Washington, DC, Baltimore, Maryland, and Birmingham, Alabama, identified evidence of previous infections among 2%–10% of the population sampled. A study in a Washington, DC, military base found that 8%–11% of patients having a febrile neurologic illness between 1941 and 1958 were seropositive for LCMV."

So sounds like LCMV epidemiologically, although patients with LCVM get leukopenia, thrombocytopenia, and mild liver function abnormalities, which he lacks. But I hate it when reality gets in the way of a good diagnosis. So I send off all the tests and...

No LCVM.

But the enteroviral PCR is positive on the spinal fluid.

Is it still enteroviral season? Barely. We have a week to go and then we can no longer wear white. Thanks to climate change, the typical 'viral meningitis' season may be changing. RSV season is shortening in England, and maybe enteroviral season is shifting as well.

An interesting case, but not what I wanted. I have yet to see a case of LCVM. But I will keep looking.

Rationalization

Lymphocytic Choriomeningitis Virus Meningitis, New York, NY, USA, 2009. https://www.ncbi.nlm.nih.gov/pmc/articles/PMC2958026/

Climate Change and the End of the Respiratory Syncytial Virus Season http://eprints.ucl.ac.uk/8004/1/8004.pdf

....

Red Bumps Redux

TODAY is kind of a repeat.

A while back I saw a case of "red bump disease" in a renal transplant infection.

The work-up had consistently yielded nothing: biopsies of the skin negative for pathogens but did have granulomas. I was sure that it was cat scratch disease, but serology was negative, as was the work up for everything else he was at risk for that can cause red bump disease in the immune-incompetent.

He was admitted for neutropenia and had a bone marrow biopsy. Nothing. The red bumps continued.

Part of the problem is that ID is such a primitive subspecialty in some ways, still relying on growing the organisms on agar, just like they did 100 years ago.

For this case, I jumped into modernity. There is a test where the 16S ribosomal sequence can be amplified from a sample of tissue, so organisms that can't be grown can be identified.

16S rRNA gene contains conserved regions useful for the design of universal PCR primers that can amplify various fragments of

the 16S rRNA gene from all pathogenic and nonpathogenic bacteria. These fragments include hypervariable regions containing species-specific signature sequences useful for bacterial identification to species level.

In other words, it's magic.

So I sent a biopsy off to the U Dub, as we call it here in Oregon, and I will be damned if they didn't find *Bartonella henselae* DNA in the tissue. He had cat scratch after all. I assume the anti-rejection medications he was on prevented a serologic response, although sero-negative illness can occur in normal people.

We demonstrated that the microorganisms existed in the cytoplasm of histiocytes within the granulomatous lesions in nine lymph nodes and one skin biopsy. Among the nine lymph nodes with IHC (+) stains, three were seronegative.

And the serology, which is usually the standard by which we make the diagnosis, is dependent on methodologies.

It is shown that the sensitivities of the IgG assays are very low (40.9% for the IFA with noncocultivated B. henselae as antigen) and that those of the IgM assays are higher (71.4% for the EIA) for patients who fulfilled two or more criteria for CSD. The IgM EIA showed the highest sensitivity: 71.4% in patients with two or more criteria for CSD and 80.6% for patients with a positive Bartonella PCR result. The results indicate that the specificities of both IFA and EIA IgG serologies and the sensitivity of the IFA IgM serology need to be improved.

Placed on a quinolone, the lesions are melting away, figuratively speaking.

Years ago my Dad told me if the tests do not support diagnosis from the history and physical, it is the test that is wrong. I need to keep that rule in mind.

Rationalization

J Formos Med Assoc. 2006 Nov;105(11):911-7. Immunohistochemical study of lymph nodes in patients with cat scratch disease. http://

www.ncbi.nlm.nih.gov/pubmed/17098692

J Clin Microbiol. 1997 Aug;35(8):1931-7. Pitfalls and fallacies of cat scratch disease serology: evaluation of Bartonella henselae-based indirect fluorescence assay and enzyme-linked immunoassay. http://www.ncbi.nlm.nih.gov/pubmed/9230358

Eur J Clin Microbiol Infect Dis. 2001 Jun;20(6):392-401. Serodiagnosis of cat scratch disease: response to Bartonella henselae in children and a review of diagnostic methods. http://www.ncbi.nlm.nih.gov/pubmed/11476439

....

Bread and Butter?

INFECTED joints are bread and butter diseases for an ID doc. No wait, that's pericarditis. What food is the infected joint? Pureed Twinkie? Curdled hollandaise? I am not certain. But infected joints are a common problem, usually due to a *Staphylococcus* or a *Streptococcus*. Usually.

Today's patient is a young female with no medical problems who comes in with 4 days of progressive pain in her knee. No past medical history, no trauma, no bacteremia- inducing procedures. The knee pain is unbearable, she is febrile, and she also has some mild right upper quadrant pain.

The exam is consistent with a septic joint and the tap shows lots of white cells but no organisms. She has elevated liver tests and an evaluation reveals her gallbladder looks bad as well. So off to the OR.

Her gallbladder is indeed inflamed and it is removed. Her knee is filled with pus and there is a surrounding soft tissue infection. The knee grows *Fusobacterium*. And *Peptostreptococcus*. And a gram negative rod that can't be identified. Her blood grows *Peptostreptococcus*. I presume she seeded her knee from the gallbladder, although the pathology shows no good reason for an acute gallbladder. No stones and, since she is from South of the border, I looked for worms and found none. Every once in a while I get called as a round worm has crawled up the common bile duct and caused obstruction. Not this time.

I have seen a smattering of mono-microbial anaerobic joint infections in my day, and it is not unheard-of.

The predominant anaerobes in arthritis are anaerobic Gram-negative bacilli (AGNB) including the Bacteroides fragilis group, Fusobacterium spp., Peptostreptococcus spp., and Propionibacterium acnes. Infection with P. acnes is associated with a prosthetic joint, previous surgery, and trauma. B. fragilis group is associated with distant infection, Clostridium spp. with trauma, and Fusobacterium spp. with oropharyngeal infection. Most cases of anaerobic arthritis, in contrast to anaerobic osteomyelitis, involved a single isolate, and most cases are secondary to hematogenous spread.

Three organisms appear to be a world's record, although the only Guinness I am likely to interact with comes in a bottle.

Unusual for infected joint, it spread into the posterior calf, a necrotizing infection that required several debridements, although by history it started in the joint.

Rationalization

J Orthop Sci. 2008 Mar;13(2):160-9. doi: 10.1007/s00776-007-1207-1. Epub 2008 Apr 8.

Microbiology and management of joint and bone <u>infections</u> due to anaerobic bacteria. <u>http://www.ncbi.nlm.nih.gov/pubmed/18392922</u>

....

Worth a Syndrome?

Six months ago I took care of a patient with pneumococcal meningitis, pneumonia and bacteremia. He received 10 days of antibiotics, and is was mostly a cure. I say "mostly" as 4 months later he came to the clinic with failure to thrive. His get up and go got up and went. Evaluation revealed a new, loud murmur. Further evaluation showed new severe mitral insufficiency on TTE but no vegetation and blood cultures were negative.

He recently had a TEE that showed a hole in the mitral valve and again no vegetations.

I think that I inadvertently treated a case of pneumococcal

endocarditis at his initial presentation, as I can think of no other reason why he would have a hole in his heart; he is not a Cindy Lauper fan.

S. pneumoniae endocarditis is uncommon; I have only seen a smattering in my career, unless, of course, I have treated a bunch without knowing it. This week I know it, as I have another case of meningitis, pneumonia and bacteremia and this time the ECHO shows a vegetation on the mitral valve.

Still unusual, I have seen no others this century. In a recent review, 2 of 136 *S. pneumoniae* bacteremias had endocarditis.

The hole in the valve is not surprising as *S. pneumoniae* is usually aggressive with

clinical characteristics of fulminant disease with frequent heart failure, complications and need for surgery

Put any three signs together, and you can have you very own syndrome: Austrian syndrome is pneumococcal pneumonia, meningitis, and endocarditis and, as a triad, is unusually reported, with about 50 cases in the literature. Not unsurprisingly, the patients do not have good outcomes. Austrian syndrome often occurs in alcoholics and while the first reported patient was not a drinker, he did have end-stage liver disease.

It was named after pneumococcal mavin Dr. Robert Austrian, not the European country, after he reported the triad in 1957. Although, does being sicker than stink from bacteria really warrant a syndrome being named after you? I don't know.

There are a lot of eponyms in medicine, although their use has been debated for years. Reiter lost his syndrome because he was a Nazi who "experimented" (it makes torture sound so benign) at the Buchenwald concentration camp.

The possessive use of an eponym should be discontinued, since the author neither had nor owned the disorder.

I still want something named after me, but I guess I'll have to catch it first.

Rationalization

Medicine (Baltimore). 2010 Sep;89(5):331-6. doi: 10.1097/
MD.0b013e3181f2b824.

The spectrum of invasive pneumococcal disease at an adult tertiary
care hospital in the early 21st century. http://www.ncbi.nlm.nih.gov/
pubmed/20827110

Int J Circumpolar Health. 2009 Sep;68(4):347-53. Endocarditis in
Greenland with special reference to endocarditis caused by Streptococcus pneumoniae. http://www.ncbi.nlm.nih.gov/pubmed/19917187

List of eponymously named diseases http://en.wikipedia.org/wiki/
List_of_eponymous_diseases

....

Associations

ID is often all about knowing associations. I have said "Give
me any situation, I will come up with a infectious disease you
can acquire as a result." Makes me fun at parties. Of course, the
smart-ass resident asked about eating Antarctic snow, and I could
not even come up with a penguin-related infection. Turns out
penguins have

> *Positive antibody titers for Chlamydophila psittaci (62%), avian
> adenovirus (7%; 1994 only), paramyxovirus-2 (7%; 1993 only),
> and Salmonella Pullorum (7%).*

But I did not know that and next time I will be ready. *Salmonella* is a good reason to make sure your penguin is cooked to at
least 160 degrees.

Every behavior and every location has an infection associated
with it. The US is not Antarctica, and, as infectious diseases go,
not all that exciting. But you still have to know what diseases are
where, or at least I need to know.

Today's patient is an elderly male on etanercept and methotrexate for rheumatoid arthritis, who visits the upper Midwest for
a long weekend and shortly after coming home has fevers, chills,
and fatigue. They get worse, with a temperature to 104, pancyto-

penia, diffuse interstitial pneumonia and hilar lymphadenopathy.

Most of the infectious work-up is negative, including a trans-bronchial biopsy of the lung. The diagnosis is thought to be lymphoma, but an astute physician (now an honorary ID doc) sends off a urine histoplasma antigen that comes back way high. A lymph node biopsy shows necrotizing granuloma and *Histoplasma*. Then they called me to treat the disseminated histoplasmosis.

There are only four common funguses/fungi you need to know about in the US: coccidiomycosis, histoplasmosis, blastomycosis and cryptococcus. And anyone on etanercept and related drugs may develop severe and/or disseminated disease with minimal exposure to these fungiuseses's. I hate the plural form of some nouns, but do like the pleural of empyema.

At the Indiana University Medical Campus (Indianapolis), 19 patients (5 children and 14 adults) have been diagnosed with histoplasmosis while receiving TNF blockers from 2000 through early 2009. Most were receiving additional immuno-suppressive agents: methotrexate in 8, azathioprine in 4, corticosteroids in 3, and 6-mercaptopurine in 1. Seventeen patients (89%) presented with progressive febrile illnesses consistent with PDH. Pulmonary involvement was present in 15 patients (79%) and was a prominent feature in 13 (68%). Thirteen cases occurred in patients who were receiving infliximab, 3 in patients who were receiving etanercept, and 3 in patients who were receiving adalimumab.

Although the study was in an endemic area, patients can have transient exposure to the dust of the Midwest and come down with histoplasmosis. All it takes is inhaling a little roadwork or other environmental dust. The air can be filled with pathogens, so do not inhale in Ohio or Indiana.

Take-home: If you have a patient on TNF inhibitors, besides the classic risk of tuberculosis, think endemic fungi, even with transient exposure. It is a rare manifestation of an unusual disease (at least in Oregon) but remember the association.

Rationalization

Arthritis Rheum. 2002 Oct;46(10):2565-70. Life-threatening histo-plasmosis complicating immunotherapy with tumor necrosis factor alpha antagonists infliximab and etanercept. http://www.ncbi.nlm.nih.gov/pubmed/12384912

Environ Health Perspect. 2005 May;113(5):585-9. Two outbreaks of occupationally acquired histoplasmosis: more than workers at risk. http://www.ncbi.nlm.nih.gov/pubmed/15866767

Clin Infect Dis. 2010 Jan 1;50(1):85-92. doi: 10.1086/648724. Rec-ognition, diagnosis, and treatment of histoplasmosis complicating tumor necrosis factor blocker therapy. http://www.ncbi.nlm.nih.gov/pubmed/19951231

....

Associations II: The Little Things

ONE of the many things that makes ID so incredibly cool is the breadth and depth of infections. ID has its tentacles in all aspects of the human condition. Sometimes it is big things, like the changing epidemiology of infections due to global warm-ing.

Sometimes it is the little things, like how the effects on sin-gle amino acid variations in the Toll-like receptors can marked-ly increase or decrease the risks of infections. Toll-like receptors (TLRs) are a class of proteins expressed on certain cells of the immune system, such as macrophages and dendritic cells. The TLRs recognize broad classes of microbial structures—bacteri-al lipoprotein, peptidoglycans, RNA, flagella, and others. When microorganisms invade the body and these structures are recog-nized, the TLRs initiate immune cell responses.

Whether you live or die from infections may depend on world-wide fossil fuel consumption or the difference between a lysine and an arginine in a protein.

My patient with the disseminated histoplasmosis is slowing improving on amphotericin, but over the last week he has devel-oped hypercalcemia—an increase in calcium. It is not due to the amphotericin, which causes potassium/magnesium wasting, but probably caused by the underlying disease.

Histoplasmosis is a disease that causes granulomas, and granulomas increase the transformation of vitamin D to 1,25-dihydroxy vitamin D. 1,25-dihydroxy vitamin D stimulates calcium absorption in the intestine as well as osteoclast-mediated calcium resorption from bone, with hypercalcemia as a consequence. Typically this is a problem with sarcoidosis, but there are a half dozen cases of hypercalcemia with disseminated histoplasmosis in humans, and one case in an owl moneky (is that a monkey or an owl?). One case was initially misdiagnosed as sarcoid.

We are aware of low vitamin D levels here in the cloudy, dark, rainy Pacific Northwest, and he has been on replacement vitamin D for low levels as an outpatient. There is also one case with the hypercalcemia in disseminated histoplasmosis exacerbated by exogenous vitamin D.

Vitamin D is perhaps more important as an immune modulator than it is for bone physiology, and it is an interesting side effect of granulomas that vitamin D production is increased.

Hypercalcemia occurs in most granulomatous disorders. High serum calcium levels are seen in about 10% of patients with sarcoidosis; hypercalciuria is about three times more frequent. Tuberculosis, fungal granulomas, berylliosis, and lymphomas are other conditions that are associated with disorders of calcium metabolism. These abnormalities of calcium metabolism are due to dysregulated production of 1,25-(OH2)D3 (calcitriol) by activated macrophages trapped in pulmonary alveoli and granulomatous inflammation.

Tuberculosis, a common cause of granuloma, is more common in vitamin D deficient people and in those with mutations in the vitamin D receptor. I wonder if the vitamin D production from granulomas is a protective result of millennia of trying to cope with tuberculosis.

1,25 Dihydroxyvitamin D3 (1,25(OH)2D3) is an important immunomodulatory hormone which activates monocytes and sup-

presses lymphocyte proliferation, immunoglobulin production and cytokine synthesis. In vitro, 1,25(OH)2D3 enhances the ability of human monocytes to restrict the growth of M. tuberculosis.

Maybe, like obesity, the metabolic effects of granulomas are a consequence of evolving with TB.

It is the little things, like vitamin D and granulomas, that may have insight into the bigger things, like human evolution. ID is so cool.

Rationalization

Am J Med. 1985 May;78(5):881-4. Hypercalcemia in disseminated histoplasmosis. Aggravation by vitamin D. http://www.ncbi.nlm.nih.gov/pubmed/3993669

BMC Infect Dis. 2010 Oct 25;10:306. doi: 10.1186/1471-2334-10-306.

Association between vitamin D insufficiency and tuberculosis in a Vietnamese population. http://www.ncbi.nlm.nih.gov/pubmed/20973965

Curr Opin Pulm Med. 2000 Sep;6(5):442-7. Hypercalcemia in granulomatous disorders: a clinical review. http://www.ncbi.nlm.nih.gov/pubmed/10958237

Genes and Immunity (2003) 4, 4–11. doi:10.1038/sj.gene.6363915. Susceptibility to mycobacterial infections: the importance of host genetics. http://www.nature.com/gene/journal/v4/n1/full/6363915a.html

JAMA. 2009 Jun 24;301(24):2586-8. doi: 10.1001/jama.2009.930.

Evolutionary speculation about tuberculosis and the metabolic and inflammatory processes of obesity. https://www.ncbi.nlm.nih.gov/pubmed/19549976

....

Threes

Do events come in threes? Of course not. Except celebrity deaths. They always occur in threes.

Had a young male with what started as a pneumonia, for which health care was not sought. Rather than improve, he worsened, and then had altered mental status. He was brought to the ER and MRI showed two early brain abscesses and a right middle lobe infiltrate on chest x-ray.

As part of the evaluation of a murmur, he had an ECHO that showed a "large 2 cm" aortic vegetation. Which is more ominous than a small 2 cm vegetation. He started sliding into heart failure as his valve fell apart and he went for quasi-emergent valve replacement, where a normal aortic valve was found, and by normal I mean there was no obvious structural abnormality to predispose the patient to endocarditis. There was a vegetation. That was not so normal.

The blood cultures? *S. pneumoniae.*

I have seen maybe one or two cases of *S. pneumoniae* endocarditis in 25 years, and I have two this month and three this year.

S. pneumoniae used to be a more common cause of endocarditis in the time before antibiotics when rheumatic fever lead to widespread valve damage.

Brain abscess? *S. pneumoniae* is even more rare as a cause of brain abscess, and the lesions on the MRI are probably infected emboli rather than true abscesses, although they do look like small enhancing pockets of pus. Of the 24 reported brain abscess from *S. pneumoniae*, only two are hematogenous, the rest being contiguous from sinusitis etc. And neither hematogenous abscesses were from endocarditis. We (the royal We, as in We are not amused) will have to follow the MRI to see if these are really abscesses (They were).

There are those books or papers that give you a conceptual framework upon which you can hang all the facts of and experience of medicine and life. For me understanding evolution was key to understanding infectious diseases. Another was *Observations on Spiraling Empiricism*, a classic that all health care providers should read, as it outlines the cognitive errors we all make in prescribing medications.

Another is T*he Drunkard's Walk: How Randomness Rules Our Lives* by Leonard Mlodinow. Events do come in threes, and twos, and fours. "Random events often come in groups/streaks/clusters," and we see a pattern where no pattern exists. Every once in a while we get a spike of healthcare-associated infections for a given quarter, but if we changed the months with which define a quarter, the spike would be occurring at a different time.

"Extraordinary events can happen without extraordinary causes," and so occasionally some poor normal patient gets aortic valve pneumococcal endocarditis. Not a satisfying answer, but the way the world often works.

Randomness, evolution, and cognitive errors. The defining characteristics of ID? It is a triad as well.

Rationalization

Clin Infect Dis. 1997 Nov;25(5):1108-12. Pyogenic brain abscess caused by Streptococcus pneumoniae: case report and review.

Am J Med. 1989 Aug;87(2):201-6. Observations on spiraling empiricism: its causes, allure, and perils, with particular reference to antibiotic therapy.

First Ever

EVERYBODY step right up and see something that no one ever has seen in the history of the this and all other universes.

Liver metastases are bad and difficult to treat. One of the therapies is to infarct the tumor. This can be done with heat or cold or, as in the case of this patient, using an intra-arterial catheter to cut off the blood supply to the tumor, killing it.

Unfortunately dead tumor is a fertile soil for bacteria and if there is a transient bacteremia from the mouth, which happens every time you brush and floss, or from the colon, which is downstream from the liver, you can get an infection.

It is rare to get an infection after arterial tumor embolization, occurring about 1.3% of the time.

Several weeks after an hepatic (a hepatic?) embolization the patient has fevers, liver pain and a marked decline in function. CT shows a big abscess in the liver which is drained and grows a pure culture of...

Here it comes, the first ever...

Streptococcus alactolyticus.

WOOT!

Ha. No human disease can be found under this name in either the Googles or the PubMeds. Finally. Something that be named after me. I hear by designate post-embolic *S. alactolyticus* liver abscess as Crislip's syndrome (tm).

What is *S. alactolyticus*? A Group D streptococcus. It is found around human teeth, the canine jejunum, and pigeon intestines. The patient has had no contact with the final two on the list.

There is a problem, of course. Streptococcal identification is not the clearest of topics. Microbiologists are always changing the classification and naming of streptococci, and it may well be that there have been other cases with this bug under a different name, but, listen up. I. Don't. Want. To. Know.

Besides, your alleged *S. alactolyticus* is as likely as not misidentified as well. I sometimes think rather than doing microbiology, the techs are collapsing wave functions get a probability answer. They tell me things like, 'It has a 80% probability of being *S. sanguis.*' I wonder if these streptococci can form an interference pattern if fired at a double slit.

But I digress. Take-home? Crislip's syndrome (tm). Popularize it and immortalize me. Better than Austrian, if you ask me.

Rationalization

Cardiovasc Intervent Radiol. 2007 Jan-Feb;30(1):6-25. http://www.
ncbi.nlm.nih.gov/pubmed/17103105. Transarterial therapy for hepa-
tocellular carcinoma: which technique is more effective? A systematic
review of cohort and randomized studies.

J Appl Microbiol. 2002;92(2):348-51. http://www.ncbi.nlm.nih.gov/
pubmed/11849364 Composition of enterococcal and streptococcal
flora from pigeon intestines.

Streptococcus alactolyticus is the dominating culturable lactic acid
bacterium species in canine jejunum and feces of four fistulated dogs.
FEMS Microbiol Lett. 2004 Jan 15;230(1):35-9. http://www.ncbi.
nlm.nih.gov/pubmed/14734163

......

First World Disease, Third World Response

THE patient is middle aged with a new diagnosis of lymphoma for which he gets rituximab and the combination chemotherapy CHOP. He is admitted with several days of shortness
of breath and ends up on a ventilator. His chest x-ray and CT
scan snow a variety of changes from long term smoking and a
ground glass infiltrate. He gets a bronchoscopy and the diagnosis
is made.

That 'P' in CHOP is the worrisome letter—it stands for prednisone. And it also stands for *Pneumocystis*, and since the former
leads to the latter, that is what the patient has.

Pneumocystis jiroveci pneumonia (PJP. note the second p is
pneumonia, so do NOT say PJP pneumonia. Or ATM machine.
Or PIN number) in the old days was primarily a disease of patients with lymphocytic malignancies who received steroids. Then
it became the most common HIV-related infection, but what is
old is new again. Thanks to HAART, I see more PJP related to
hematologic malignancies and the newer therapies for rheuma-
tologic diseases.

Whether rituximab is a risk factor for PJP is uncertain, there
are cases reports, and association is not causation, although

whacking your remaining T cells can't be all that helpful for the immune system.

The treatment of choice for PJP has been and remains trimethoprim/ sulfamethoxazole (TMP/Sulfa). All the other therapies have higher failure rates, more toxicities, or both. TMP/ Sulfa resistance has been reported and is due to mutations of the dihydropteroate synthase gene, the binding site of the drug. As a rule resistance occurs in patients who have been on long-term prophylaxis, so this patient should not be at risk.

One wonders, and that one is me, that with the increased use of TMP/Sulfa to treat MRSA, what antibiotic pressure we are putting on *Pneumocystis*, which is part of our normal flora. There is data to suggest that the organism is spread person to person, including resistant strains.

So one of the consequences of MRSA may be more *Pneumocystis* resistance.

However, I practice in the US, where the care is second to none, so I put the patient on IV TMP/Sulfa and he got... What? There is not any IV TMP/Sulfa in the US? You must be kidding. We have the best health care in the world, how could we be out of a critical antibiotic? Does Cuba have any they could lend us?

I cannot find the reason why TMP/Sulfa is no longer available. Probably because one company makes it and there is something wrong with the one factory that produces the stuff. This is not unusual; we had a nitroglycerine shortage when a hurricane shut down the plant in Puerto Rico.

There is stable equilibrium, where a ball sits in the bottom of a glass. There is unstable equilibrium, where a ball sits on top of an overturned glass. It seems like our health care "system" more often than not resembles the latter. But at least I can get my patients all the erectile dysfunction meds they need so they can die happy.

Rationalization

Acta Haematol. 2010;123(1):30-3. doi: 10.1159/000261020. Epub 2009 Nov 25. Granulomatous Pneumocystis jiroveci pneumonia in a patient with diffuse large B-cell lymphoma: case report and review of the literature. http://www.ncbi.nlm.nih.gov/pubmed/19940467

J Chin Med Assoc. 2008 Nov;71(11):579-82. doi: 10.1016/S1726-4901(08)70173-4. Pneumocystis jiroveci pneumonia in patients with non-Hodgkin's lymphoma receiving chemotherapy containing rituximab.

http://www.ncbi.nlm.nih.gov/pubmed/19015057

Hurricane Georges Causes Shortage Of Nitroglycerin Tablet In U.S. http://boards.medscape.com/forums/.29f3af03/!discloc=.2a04b-5f7&nopopup=1

....

Numbers

I LIKE numbers. What is the importance of *"Formate assay in body fluids: application in methanol poisoning?"* It is the first entry in PubMed. #1. The millionth? *"DNA- and RNA-dependent DNA polymerases: progressive changes in rabbit endometrium during preimplantation stage of pregnancy."* The ten millionth? *"Optical properties of excitons under an axial-potential perturbation."*

The 666th? Curiously, it's *"Patient Acceptance of an Electronic Subcutaneous Identifier."*

Not really.

It is *Urinary acidification in renal allografts.* Put a random, or semi-random number into PubMed and get a result. My birthday yields *"The role of estradiol in experimental parasitosis caused by* Schistosoma mansoni *in the female golden hamster* Cricetus auratus." Probably not significant.

Numbers are sometimes meaningless, sometimes not. Take 35. Often bad if it's your diastolic blood pressure, respiratory rate, temperature and white blood cell count, as is the case in this patient. He started with what looked like zoster, then developed fevers and rigors. Over the next 12 hours he acutely decompensated and ended up in the ICU on a ventilator.

The physical exam showed a smattering of small pustules all over his body in addition to the zoster and a red, hot, swollen sternoclavicular (SC) joint. The CT of the chest showed multiple round lesions throughout the lung, but the transthoracic echocardiography (TTE) was negative for vegetations that would suggest endocarditis. My bet was htat the reason the TTE was negative was all the clot was downstream in the lung, plus the usual increased patient size that makes a TTE hard to read. All the blood cultures grew methicillin sensitive *Staphylococcus aureus* (MSSA).

I think the patient has Varicella-zoster virus with disseminated zoster and the skin lesions allowed access of MSSA to his bloodstream that seeded his valve and SC joint. When patients get shingles it is not that uncommon to get a few pox elsewhere. It is less common to get right sided endocarditis. Like no reported cases.

Zoster and secondary infections go together, although the secondaries are usually Group A streptococcus, sometimes with necrotizing fasciitis. A risk may be the use of NSAIDS. I suppose the anti-inflammatory effect of the NSAID tilts the battle in the favor the group A streptococcus. It may not be causal, but it is a worry. Because this patient was on a ventilator, I couldn't ask him if took any NSAIDs. I found out later that he did not.

Staphylococcus is seen less often with cutaneous zoster, or at least less often reported. Given how *Staphylococcus* likes to invade damaged skin, it would be like reporting water is wet or ice is cold.

Rationalization

Clin Exp Dermatol. 1998 Mar;23(2):87-8. Necrotizing fasciitis complicating disseminated cutaneous herpes zoster.

Clin Exp Dermatol. 2008 May;33(3):249-55. Epub 2008 Feb 2. Severe necrotizing soft-tissue infections and nonsteroidal anti-inflammatory drugs.

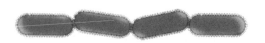

Why Is ID Different?

WE are heading into *Salmonella* season, er, I mean Thanksgiving, and as is the case around the holidays, the hospital slows down. No one wants to risk having to eat hospital turkey and pumpkin pie for Thanksgiving. So I will rant on a peripheral topic.

No one would ever change the dialysis orders in a renal patient, or the ventilator settings on a pulmonary patient, or alter the chemotherapy on an oncology patient. But, it seems, people seem to have no problem changing antibiotics on a patient with an ID consult.

Lest you think this is all about me and is the just deserts for an arrogant dumbass, I was talking with a colleague who was wondering what to do when docs change around his antibiotics and do not even have the courtesy to call him. Not long ago one of the University docs made a similar complaint. This used to happen to me, but less as the years go by. With age comes some authority, and it has been a while since anyone has messed with my orders. And I encourage the medicine residents to make decisions when I am not around; we can discuss the pros and cons later. It is always a learning experience to be wrong.

But what is it about antibiotics and infections? People who really have no idea what they are doing feel free to change things around, and more often than not, for the worse. I am not talking about issues where reasonable people may differ, like the best treatment for MRSA pneumonia. I am talking about issues where it is reasonably clear what the best therapy is: MSSA bacteremia or Group A streptococcus soft tissue infection. And, it seems, the farther the doc is from ID, the more likely they are going to alter my antibiotics. A subspecialty surgeon is far more likely to change my antibiotics than a hospitalist.

I have two theories, and perhaps you will offer others.

The first is that for most people infections are more akin to demons and antibiotics more akin to spells. Most health care providers do not think in terms of microbiology and pharmacology.

They think there is an evil bug that must be killed with a big gun—some powerful, strong drug. I have said for years that it is 100% sensitive and specific that anyone who uses the terms 'big gun,' 'powerful,' or 'strong' about antibiotics knows nothing, literally zero, about treating infections. They have been suckered into using advertising terms and can't be trusted. They probably think that a close shave will result in a pretty girl rubbing the back of her hand against their cheek.

The other option, and the two are not mutually exclusive, is the Dunning–Kruger effect.

Kruger and Dunning proposed that, for a given skill, incompetent people will:

- tend to overestimate their own level of skill;

- fail to recognize genuine skill in others;

- fail to recognize the extremity of their inadequacy;

- recognize and acknowledge their own previous lack of skill, if they can be trained to substantially improve.

The Dunning–Kruger effect is a cognitive bias in which an unskilled person makes poor decisions and reaches erroneous conclusions, but their incompetence denies them the metacognitive ability to realize their mistakes. The unskilled therefore suffer from illusory superiority, rating their own ability as above average, much higher than it actually is, while the highly skilled underrate their abilities, suffering from illusory inferiority. This leads to the situation in which less competent people rate their own ability higher than more competent people. It also explains why actual competence may weaken self-confidence: because competent individuals falsely assume that others have an equivalent understanding.

The Dunning–Kruger effect, combined with the Peter Principle, does explain so much.

But don't mess with my antibiotics.

Rationalization

Dunning–Kruger effect

http://en.wikipedia.org/wiki/Dunning%E2%80%93Kruger_effect

Peter principle: http://en.wikipedia.org/wiki/Peter_Principle

....

Coke Adds Life

MY patient with the disseminated histoplasmosis has done phenomenally well. After a month on amphotericin his histoplasma antigen went from 36 to zero, and clinically he has done well. It is always fun to see people go from sicker than stink to mostly normal with time and antibiotics. I do not know exactly what the look is that really ill people have, but I know it when I see it. And one day, poof, the look is gone and now when you look into the patient's eyes there is someone home.

It's time for oral therapy, so I have put him on itraconazole with Coke.

Coke you ask? Yes. The cola.

Itraconazole requires acid for absorption, and Coke is acidic. The elderly are often hypochlorhydric as well, not to mention all the ways we have in medicine to increase stomach pH. So a little Coke may help.

RESULTS: Serum itraconazole concentrations, after administration with Coca-Cola (treatment II), were higher than after administration with water (treatment I). The mean AUC was 1.12 vs 2.02 micrograms.h.m1-1, the mean Cmax was 0.14 vs 0.31 micrograms.m1-1 and the mean tmax was 2.56 vs 3.38 h in treatments I and II, respectively.

CONCLUSION: The absorption of itraconazole can be enhanced by Coca-Cola.

and

An analysis of the area under the curve (AUC) and peak plasma concentration (Cmax) data indicated that the bioavailability of itraconazole was significantly reduced when the gastric pH was increased by pretreatment with ranitidine but showed that this effect was counteracted by the coadministration of an acidic solution (e.g., a cola beverage) that transiently reduced the gastric pH. These findings suggest that the coadministration of an acidic beverage with itraconazole may be an effective approach in improving the bioavailability of itraconazole in patients who are hypochlorhydric or who are taking gastric acid suppressants.

Other drinks?

Coadministration of grapefruit juice did not affect any pharmacokinetic parameter of itraconazole while that of orange juice decreased the parameters of T1/2, AUC, and AUC/S of the drug.

No data with beer, although the pH of most beers is between 3.90 and 4.20. Other sodas?

Coke pH was 2.44, Pepsi pH was 2.46, Dr. Pepper pH was 2.93, Sprite pH was 2.88, Moutain Dew pH was 3.23, and Mug root beer pH was 4.06.

So they should all work, although the published data is with Coke.

Less clear is when to stop the itraconazole. He may need methotrexate and a TNF-inhibitor again in the future, and can I guarantee a cure? No. Should the itraconazole be for life? Or restarted when he starts immunosuppressants?

The guidelines say

Lipid formulation of amphotericin B (3.0–5.0 mg/kg daily intravenously for 1–2 weeks) followed by itraconazole (200 mg 3 times daily for 3 days and then 200 mg twice daily, for a total of 12 weeks)." and that "lifelong suppressive therapy may be useful in patients with other immunosuppressive disorders in whom immunosuppression cannot be substantially reduced.

The patient is off immunosuppressive meds currently, but in the future? Who knows.

"When it comes to the future, there are three kinds of people: those who let it happen, those who make it happen, and those who wonder what happened." —John M. Richardson, Jr.

In medicine I try to take the middle option. Probably itraconazole for life.

Rationalization

Eur J Clin Pharmacol. 1997;52(3):235-7. Influence of an acidic beverage (Coca-Cola) on the absorption of itraconazole. http://www.ncbi.nlm.nih.gov/pubmed/9218932

J Clin Pharmacol. 1997 Jun;37(6):535-40. Effect of a cola beverage on the bioavailability of itraconazole in the presence of H2 blockers. http://www.ncbi.nlm.nih.gov/pubmed/9208361

Int J Clin Pharmacol Ther. 1998 Jun;36(6):306-8. Effect of grapefruit juice on pharmacokinetics of itraconazole in healthy subjects. http://www.ncbi.nlm.nih.gov/pubmed/9660036

Clinical Infectious Diseases 2007;45:807–825. Clinical Practice Guidelines for the Management of Patients with Histoplasmosis: 2007 Update by the Infectious Diseases Society of America http://www.journals.uchicago.edu/doi/full/10.1086/521259

Negative

I LIKE to be an upbeat, positive kind of guy. For me, the glass is not only half full, it is half full of unicorn smiles. But sometimes life gives you lemons and you can't always make a lemon chiffon pie.

The patient is an elderly male who has been ill for an uncertain period of time; per the family he has been ill three or four days prior to admission. He is found incoherent and brought into the hospital.

He has fevers, a heart murmur, widespread pulmonary emboli, leukocytosis, thrombocytopenia. Echocardiography shows large vegetations on both the mitral and tricuspid valves of the heart. He has what looks to be renal failure from glomerular nephritis.

So the history suggests acute infection, and with all the emboli I would expect *S. aureus.*

From the size and location of the vegetations, combined with a disease of sufficient duration to cause glomerular nephritis, I expect a more chronic cause of endocarditis.

And the cultures grow: nothing.

Zip. Zilch. Nil.

So it is a case of culture-negative endocarditis. Is it culture-negative due to prior treatment with antibiotics? No. The patient doesn't see doctors. Could it be a fastidious organism like *Abiotrophia* that's difficult to see on culture plates? If so, it is really fastidious. Multiple cultures are all negative.

Maybe it's one of the organisms we can't grow at all? I send for serologies for everything that can be tested. All negative. I look for tumor and collagen vascular disease. Big fat nothing.

Non-infectious causes of culture-negative endocarditis occur in about 2.5% of patients. Infectious causes are reported in a huge series and are as follows:

Table 5

Comparison of Microorganisms Identified in Published Series of Blood Culture–Negative Endocarditis

Microorganism	Present study[a] (n = 740)	Study by location [reference]			
		France [3] (n = 348)	France [29] (n = 88)	Great Britain [30] (n = 63)	Algeria [31] (n = 62)
Bartonella species	12.4	28.4	0	9.5	22.6
Brucella melitensis	0	0	0	0	1.6
Chlamydia species	0	0	2.2	1.6	0
Corynebacterium species	0.5	0	1.1	0	1.6
Coxiella burnetii	37.0	48	7.9	12.7	3.2
Enterobacteriaceae	0.5	0	0	0	0
HACEK bacteria	0.5	0	0	0	3.2
Staphylococcus species	2.0	0	3.4	11.1	6.4
Streptococcus species	4.4	0	1.1	6.3	3.2
Tropheryma whipplei	2.6	0.3	0	0	0
Other bacteria	3.0	1.1	1.1	1.6	1.6
Fungi	1.0	0	0	6.3	1.6
No etiology	36.5	22.1	82.9	50.8	54.8

NOTE. Data are percentages. HACEK, *Haemophilus, Actinobacillus, Cardiobacterium, Eikenella, Kingella.*

[a] Patients classified as excluded were not included in this analysis.

The common causes are

"Chronic Q fever (IgG titer to phase I C. burnetii, >1:800) was diagnosed in 274 patients (77%). Eighty patients (22.5%) had an IgG titer to B. quintana and/or B. henselae 1:800"

as well as a smattering of other organisms.

What does he have? Probably will not know unless we take the valve out and send the tissue to the University of Washington for broad spectrum analysis using polymerase chain reaction (PCR). But he is not amenable to surgical intervention.

So I will probably never know. At least he is slowly getting better on antibiotics.

Update: He got better and so we never had a diagnosis.

Rationalization

Clinical Infectious Diseases 2010;51:131–140. Comprehensive Diagnostic Strategy for Blood Culture–Negative Endocarditis: A Prospective Study of 819 New Cases. http://www.journals.uchicago.edu/doi/full/10.1086/653675

Hemoptysis

Everyone can cough up a little blood with a bad case of bronchitis. However, 350 cc? I don't think in metric very well, so I have to convert it to a measurement I understand. That is 8.93 drams! That's a lot of blood.

The patient is a young homeless male with an alcohol habit.

The chest x-ray and CT scam both show bilateral upper lobe consolidation/cavities/scarring and his smear is positive for acid-fast bacilli, the family of organisms that includes the causative agent of tuberculosis. TB or not TB, that is the question; cultures are pending.

Hemoptysis is a classic complication of TB, and fortunately the patient's bleeding stopped on its own and the CT angiogram found nothing to embolize. About a decade ago we had a patient with refractory bleeding from TB who eventually died as his lungs filled up with bleeding that we could not stop. Unbelievably awful.

Why the huge bleeding with TB? The common cause is a Rasmussen's aneurysm—an aneurysm of the pulmonary artery, which sits adjacent to or within a cavity and then ruptures. Rasmussen's aneurysm occurs in about 5% of patients with TB and is in a hard place to put a bandaid on; the usual treatment is embolization. I always remember, perhaps incorrectly, that Sonia's stepmother in *Crime and Punishment* had TB, and they treated her hemoptysis with bleeding. Always seemed counterproductive.

A wee bit of anti-tubercular antibiotics and the patient will be OK. I hope. The patient is from Micronesia where they have had two clusters of multi drug resistant (MDR) TB.

These two clusters of MDR TB represent two distinct outbreaks and illustrate two mechanisms for the emergence of drug resis-

tance. In the first outbreak, the index patient had not been treated previously for TB and probably became infected with a MDR TB strain before returning to Chuuk in 2000 from Saipan; this case illustrates primary (i.e., initial) drug resistance. In the second outbreak, lack of DOT for the five family members with TB disease initially resistant to only isoniazid and ethionamide probably led to secondary (i.e., acquired) rifampin resistance. At least one of these five previous patients thus acquired multidrug resistance and transmitted MDR TB to the index case in the second outbreak.

Per the *Morbidity and Mortality Weekly Report*, Micronesia is not the best place to get TB:

FSM comprises four states and more than 600 islands spread across 1 million square miles in the western Pacific Ocean. Half of the population of 108,000 lives in Chuuk, the largest state (2). TB is endemic in Chuuk, where 70 cases of TB were recorded in 2007. The 2007 incidence rate (127 TB cases per 100,000) is 29 times higher than the 2007 U.S. rate (3). Limited transportation hinders access to the only hospital in Chuuk, which provides chest radiography and smear microscopy services to help diagnose TB. Culture confirmation, drug-susceptibility testing, and genotyping were not available routinely for TB cases in FSM until January 2006, when referral laboratories in Hawaii and California began to offer these services. Before 2008, the state's geography, combined with limited TB program staffing, precluded active case-finding via routine contact investigations or the administration of DOT, a cornerstone of TB treatment that improves completion of therapy and prevents the emergence of drug resistance. Before July 2008, TB patients were identified as they showed signs or symptoms of TB disease at the local clinic or hospital; all received self-administered therapy. FSM's National TB Program has an annual budget of $170,000, and second-line drugs for treating MDR TB were not available because of funding constraints.

Evidently there is a special relationship, a Compact of Free Association, between Micronesia and the US where its citizens can, under some circumstances, come to the US without a visa and as a result may not get the usual infectious disease screening.

They also advise against heavy drinking and public drunkenness as the US is "much more disapproving" of such behavior, as well as of rape and violence towards women. They party hearty in Micronesia.

Rationalization

Rasmussen's Aneurysm http://www.nejm.org/doi/full/10.1056/NE-JMicm050783

Rasmussen's aneurysm — undue importance to an uncommon entity? http://bjr.birjournals.org/cgi/content/full/82/980/698

Two Simultaneous Outbreaks of Multidrug-Resistant Tuberculosis —- Federated States of Micronesia, 2007—2009.http://www.cdc.gov/MMWR/preview/mmwrhtml/mm5810a3.htm

Compact of Free Association. http://en.wikipedia.org/wiki/Compact_of_Free_Association

ESSENTIAL INFORMATION FOR CITIZENS OF THE FEDERATED STATES OF MICRONESIA TRAVELING TO THE UNITED STATES AND POSSESSIONS. http://www.pireport.org/articles/2002/07/12/essential-information-citizens-federated-states-micronesia-traveling-united

....

Never Heard Of It

I HAVE been out of medical school and in the mines of medicine for 27 years. That's a long time, more than half my life. I have easily seen 29 thousand patients or more in my career, in one capacity or another. Yet, day after day I see diseases I have never seen before. Internal Medicine and Infectious Diseases appears almost infinite in the ability to deliver up new (to me) diseases. When people marvel at human physiology and its abilities, I see the innumerable ways we can go bad.

The patient is in her mid-forties and presents with a new encephalopathy, some agitation that progresses to coma.

The MRI scan of her brain and lumbar puncture (LP), are

negative but an electroencephalogram (EEG) shows persistent subacute seizures. They call me and neurology.

I do not find a reason for infection: no history, physical, or lab findings to suggest a disease in my bailiwick expect for fevers, and she is having documented aspiration as a potential cause of the fevers. In favor of aspiration is that she needs intubation for airway protection, and the fevers abate after the tube is placed.

So she is young, has a coma, seizures, was encephalopathic before she went into coma and the best I can say is that she it is probably not due to an infectious disease.

Neurology sends off, of all things, thyroid studies and she is hypothyroid with an extremely elevated thyroid peroxidase antibody.

The patient has Hashimoto's thyroiditis and there is an associated encephalitis, an extremely rare disease with about 200 cases in the literature.

It is

...a controversial neurological disorder that comprises a heterogenous group of neurological symptoms that manifest in patients with high titers of antithyroid antibodies. Clinical manifestations of HE may include encephalopathic features such as seizures, behavioral and psychiatric manifestations, movement disorders, and coma. Although it has been linked to cases of Hashimoto's thyroiditis or thyroid dysfunction, the most common immunological feature of HE is the presence of high titers of antithyroglobulin or anti-TPO (antimicrosomal) antibodies. At present, it is unclear whether antithyroid antibodies represent an immune epiphenomenon in a subset of patients with encephalopathic processes or they are really associated with pathogenic mechanisms of the disorder.

She fits the clinical diagnosis although there is little known about the pathophysiology. There seem, for example, to be no cross-reacting antibodies between the thyroid and the brain to account for the disease.

Score one for neurology. I hate being aced by another service.

She is on steroids, which is the treatment, and we will see if she improves.

Another odd cause of encephalopathy. About five years ago we had a case of an agitated encephalopathy in a young female that was due to a teratoma. Teratomas are weird tumors that can have all sorts of mature tissue in it: brain, teeth and hair for the example. In that disease there are antibodies directed against the brain tissue in the teratoma that also react with the neurons in the limbic system of the brain, another weird cause of an encephalitis that is not infectious. I did not make that diagnosis either.

There is an old medical joke that you make the diagnosis of a teratoma with "cryo-auscultation": put the patient in a cold room then listen in the abdomen to see if you can hear teeth chattering. Yeah, medical humor can be odd.

Maybe if I am in practice another 27 years I will see another of each. So much to see, so little time.

Update: She got better with the steroids.

___

Rationalization

CNS Drugs. 2007;21(10):799-811. Hashimoto's encephalopathy : epidemiology, pathogenesis and management. http://www.ncbi.nlm.nih.gov/pubmed/17850170

http://onlinelibrary.wiley.com/doi/10.1196/annals.1444.018/abstract

Paraneoplastic anti–N-methyl-D-aspartate receptor encephalitis associated with ovarian teratoma. http://onlinelibrary.wiley.com/doi/10.1002/ana.21050/full

Why I Am Not Upset When Bambi's Mother Is Shot

ODAY's patient has flu-like symptoms.

What are flu-like symptoms for this patient? He reports nausea and vomiting. Not what I consider the flu, and it is rare for a patient to report a febrile, myalgia, coughing syndrome as due to the flu. It is odd that most flu-like symptoms, from the patient's perspective, are rarely from influenza. Flu is identified as a "coughing illness," not flu-like symptoms. Wonder why.

Shortly after the nausea and vomiting, he experiences increasing pain in his hip to the point where he cannot walk and he goes to the ER. A tap of the joint shows 33,000 white blood cells, all polymorphonuclear leucocytes or "polys," and no organisms. He is off to the OR for debridement.

The surgeon tells me it was PID (pus in dere, an old joke from my Minnesota residency, oh yeah sure don't cha know), and the gram stain shows a few gram positive cocci and cultures remain negative.

When I see the patient he has no risk factors for a septic hip. None. He is a student, no trauma, no other infection, no family history, no animal exposure and his exam is negative for any other pathology.

However, he is new to the great Pacific Northwest, having just moved here from Maine, land of the faux Portland.

So I ask Lyme questions.

Any rashes, other joint problems, neurologic or heart issues? None.

He did work in a park that, he informs me, is Lyme central since they cannot hunt in the park and the deer population is taking off. One of his coworkers had Lyme.

And a quick Google informs me that Lyme rates are taking off in Maine.

And I will be damned if his Lyme serology isn't positive as is the confirmatory Western Blot.

We have almost no Lyme in Oregon, and the real cases I have seen have been imported from the Northeast. I once had a patient with bilateral due to Lyme in a kid who was from Old Lyme, Connecticut. It wasn't a hard diagnosis to make once you had a travel history. I do not think I would live in a city named Syphilis or SmallPox, much less Old Lyme. Seems to be tempting fate.

It would appear from the literature that the hip is a distinctly odd joint for Lyme involvement. Synovitis is far more common than an acute inflammatory hip.

In favor of Lyme: culture negative, no reason for a septic hip, he has a positive serology from an endemic area.

Against Lyme: gram positive cocci on the gram stain (which after review were not impressive and could be artifact; gram stains are not as clear cut as one would like) and the hip involvement.

So I will treat him for both, killing two stones with one bird.

I hope my readers from Lyme endemic areas will comment on the hip manifestations of Lyme and enlighten this inexperienced Oregonian.

Rationalization

Clin Orthop Relat Res. 1993 Jan;(286):212-4. Acute arthritis of the hip in a child infected with the Lyme spirochete. http://www.ncbi. nlm.nih.gov/pubmed/8425348

Lyme disease could soar this year. http://www.pressherald.com/news/ lyme-disease-could-soar-this-year_2010-04-04.html

But Wait. There's More

ARE you an Occam's kind of guy, or a Hickam's kind of gal? I trend to the Occam's side of the razor and like to have a unifying diagnosis for the symptoms. In the old days AIDS patients were the one group of patients where Occam's razor never worked.

Patients, in the pre-HAART era, would present with multiple infections. Now, it would seem, Rituxan et al. and steroids are acting as the moral (immoral? amoral?) equivalent of old school AIDS. Both suppress the immune system; Rituxan (brand name for Rituximab) is an antibody against CD20. Since CD20 is primarily found on immune system B cells, this drug targets B cells and gives relief from autoimmune conditions and some forms of cancer—but also leaves the patient vulnerable to infection.

The patient is an elderly male on high dose dexamethasone and Rituxan for refractory idiopathic thromobocytopenic purpura. He does not even have a lymphocyte-related malignancy. After a month of dexamethasone the platelets are better but within a week of stopping the dexamethasone the patient develops rapid and progressive shortness of breath.

A chest X-ray shows diffuse bilateral infiltrates and a bronchoscopy shows *Pneumocystis jiroveci* pneumonia (PJP). No surprise—just like the old AIDS days.

Here is a pearl for you, and, given my odd grammar, a perl.

For non-AIDS patients on steroids, they get symptomatic PJP AFTER the steroids are withdrawn. What is presumably occurring is that the *Pneumocystis* multiplies in the lung while the patient is on steroids, then when the 'roids are withdrawn, the white blood cells invade to kill the PJP and cause inflammation and symptoms. It is kinda sorta an Immune Reconstitution Inflammatory Syndrome.

But wait. There's more.

The bronchoscopy also had lots of white cells and "4 plus" gram positive rods. The real deal? Maybe. First they say it is a *Corynebacterium*. Well, some *Corynebacterium* cause pneumonia, so maybe it is a cause of disease, and the next day the lab calls it *C. pseudodiphtheriticum*. That's a pulmonary pathogen, and there is one case with *C. pseudodiphtheriticum* causing simultaneous disease with PJP in an AIDS patient. This is, if memory serves, the second *C. pseudodiphtheriticum* in my career.

So the patient has two diseases.

But wait, there's more.

Well, kind of.

The bronchoscopy grew scant *Candida*, which never ever never ever and never never causes pneumonia and can be safely ignored. And a few *Aspergillus*, which I will cautiously ignore, since the CT scan of the chest showed no cavities.

But wait. There's even more. Could that be a cavity on the scan?

Certainly no cavity that could be seen. But the patient did develop a pneumothorax, a complication we did see with regularity in the bad old days when we called PJP PCP. PCP leads to

Subpleural necrosis with bleb formation as well as bullous changes persisted even in the absence of an alveolar filling process. We conclude that the mechanism for pneumothorax in PCP is spon-

taneous rupture of necrotic lung tissue occurring in a subgroup of AIDS patients in which the interstitial inflammatory response to Pneumocystis has been accelerated.

With the relatively rapid onset and progression of shortness of breath after the steroids were stopped, I suspect that this patient also had an accelerated inflammatory response that led to a necrotic bleb and a popped lung— aka the pneumothorax. If pneumothorax has been described in non-HIV PJP, I can't find it on PubMed. I am not so good with the Boolean NOTS; for me they are Gordian knots.

So much pathology in one patient, it is hard to stick with Occam in the era of Rituxan.

But wait. There's more.

Not really. No free shipping, no steak knives, no slap chop, no 1-800 number to call. I'm done for today.

Rationalization

Diagn Microbiol Infect Dis. 1999 Apr;33(4):209-16.Corynebacterium pseudodiphtheriticum: an easily missed respiratory pathogen in HIV-infected patient. http://www.ncbi.nlm.nih.gov/pubmed/10212746

Clin Infect Dis. 1995 Jan;20(1):37-40. Corynebacterium pseudodiphtheriticum: a respiratory tract pathogen in adults. http://www.ncbi.nlm.nih.gov/pubmed/7727667

Recurrent pneumothorax in AIDS patients with Pneumocystis pneumonia. A clinicopathologic report of three cases and review of the literature. http://chestjournal.chestpubs.org/content/98/2/266

Occam's razor: The principle can be interpreted as stating Among competing hypotheses, the one with the fewest assumptions should be selected. https://en.wikipedia.org/wiki/Occam's_razor.

Hickam's dictum is a counterargument to the use of Occam's razor in the medical profession. The principle is commonly stated: "Patients can have as many diseases as they damn well please". https://en.wikipedia.org/wiki/Hickam%27s_dictum

Where The Bug Refuses To Die

I LIKE to kill. Bacteria, fungi, parasites—viruses maybe not so much. Can you kill the undead? A virus has no brain to put a bullet in. Rick Grimes of *The Walking Dead* has it easy. If there is karma for causing death in this life, I am doomed in the next, for I am directly responsible for the deaths of billions upon billions of organisms. And when they don't die? That's a failure.

Today I encounter a middle-aged dialysis patient (fistula, not catheter) who has a coagulase-negative staphylococcal bacteremia. She is placed on vancomycin and, while afebrile, her blood cultures are persistently positive on day 3. And day 7. And day 14. And day 20. According to the standard sensitivity pattern the organism is only susceptible to vancomycin, with a minimal inhibitory concentration (MIC) of 1.0. Her vancomycin levels are fine and she has an ECHO that shows aortic valve endocarditis. She is transferred to my hospital for valve replacement for failure of antibiotics. At my institution the blood cultures are again positive in less than 24 hours for the same damn staph.

Health-care-related, coagulase-negative staphylococcus endocarditis is not such a benign disease for such relatively non-un-a-pathogenic organism, with mortality equal to *S. aureus* endocarditis. Methicillin-resistant strains are particularly deadly.

In turn, NVE (native valve endocarditis) caused by methicillin-resistant CoNS [coagulase-negative staphylococci] was associated with significantly higher rates of persistent bacteremia (25 versus 9%; P = 0.01) and in-hospital mortality (40 versus 16%; P = 0.03) than methicillin-susceptible isolates.

Which is always the case. Compared to beta-lactams, all antibiotics stink on ice for staphylococi. I suppose he could have a heteroresistant Staphylococcus.

Heteroresistant vancomycin-intermediate Staphylococcus aureus (hetero-VISA) strains are those for which MICs are conventional (≤4 μg/ml) except when high-density inocula are used; with such inocula, there are minority subpopulations for which MICs are in the intermediate range (8 to 16 μg/ml)

None of the blood cultures are growing organisms with higher MICs in this case.

Before she gets a new valve I make sure, as best as we can, that there is no other source for bacteremia and none is found, and I change her, with not much enthusiasm, to daptomycin. Repeat blood cultures are negative after 48 hours. Finally I am the Bringer of Death—which, oddly, is a rare staff.

But now what?

Daptomycin is not usually used for left-sided endocarditis, and there is exactly one case like mine where daptomycin was used successfully. Not a great deal of data upon which to base a decision.

So far so good, but given the propensity for daptomycin resistance to occur in *S. aureus* while on therapy, I am worried this is the calm before the storm. She will need a valve for hemodynamic reasons, but sooner or later? Got me.

Follow-up: The daptomycin worked.

Rationalization

Ann Clin Microbiol Antimicrob. 2010 Feb 18;9:9. Daptomycin for methicillin-resistant Staphylococcus epidermidis native-valve endocarditis: a case report. http://www.ncbi.nlm.nih.gov/pubmed/20167084

Braz J Infect Dis. 2007 Jun;11(3):345-50. Heterogeneous resistance to vancomycin and teicoplanin among Staphylococcus spp. isolated from bacteremia. http://www.ncbi.nlm.nih.gov/pubmed/176846

J Clin Microbiol. 2005 May; 43(5): 2494–2496. Unstable Vancomycin Heteroresistance Is Common among Clinical Isolates of Methicillin-Resistant Staphylococcus aureus. http://www.ncbi.nlm.nih.gov/pmc/articles/PMC1153753/

One More Thing I Do Not Miss From the Old Days

You young whippersnappers do not know how lucky you have it. Back in the day when you wanted to find a new piece of information to answer a question, you had to go to the *Index Medicus*. Every year, in teeny tiny print, every title—but not the abstract, so you never knew if it was worth reading—was published in a huge series about the size of the World Book Encyclopedia. The only way you could get to the library was barefoot, up hill through the snow. You had to slowly go through each year's volume, copy the reference, go to the stack, pull the article and see if it applied to your question. It usually didn't, so you went through the process, rinse lather repeat, until you found a reference that answered your question.

Today I saw a patient with maybe pneumonia. She had a smoking history and grew MRSA out of her sputum last admission, but the odd thing was the series of chest X-rays. She had some patchy infiltrates but no real consolidation and was never really all that ill.

She was readmitted with increased shortness of breath while on oral clindamycin for her pneumonia. We discovered she had developed at large, multiloculated pleural effusion that was treated with a video-assisted thoracoscopic surgery. Gram stain and white blood cell count from the surgery were negative and they called me.

For reasons that are too painful to mention, other studies on the pleural fluid were not done: lactate dehydrogenase, pH, and so on, which would tell us if it's a transudate or an exudate. So while it doesn't look like an empyema, or pus in the chest cavity, by gram stain, I can't say with certainly since I lack the data.

The CT scan of the chest not only showed mutiloculated fluid, but no rim enhancement as one would expect with empyema, and there was numerous small 1 cm (different than large 1 cm) mediastinal and hilar lymph nodes. Is it, I wonder, tumor, like lymphoma? The loculation on CT suggests high protein in the fluid, and there was not the consolidation in the lung parenchyma you would expect to result in a complicated parapneumonic effusion.

I am discussing the case with the resident and ask, not knowing the answer, "how often do you see lymphadenopathy with community acquired pneumonia?"

He didn't know either, so I turned to PubMed while he raced me using the Googles.

And in less than a minute we had found "*The characteristics and significance of thoracic lymphadenopathy in parapneumonic effusion and empyema.*"

And the answer?

The appearances of mediastinal lymph nodes were recorded in 50 consecutive patients with parapneumonic effusion/empyema. 18 (36%) had mediastinal lymphadenopathy (node size greater than 1 cm). The mean number of enlarged nodes was 1.9 (range 1-3) and the mean size was 1.4 cm (2 cm maximum). Seven patients had a single involved site, nine patients two sites and two patients three sites. The right paratracheal area was most commonly involved and the subcarinal area contained the largest nodes. The presence of enlarged nodes did not correlate with biochemical and microbiological stage of pleural infection, length of history, or extent of consolidation. This study shows that mediastinal lymphadenopathy is commonly associated with parapneumonic effusion and that multiple sites may be involved. The degree of enlargement is moderate although lymphadenopathy of greater than 2 cm size should raise the possibility of other pathology.

So it would appear that there is a wee bit more adenopathy by numbers but not by size than one would except for a community acquired pneumonia, so maybe this is malignant. We are getting more pleural fluid to see.

That answer, found at light speed, would have taken the better part of an afternoon when I was a fellow and we wore onions on our belt as was the style of the day.

You do not know how lucky you have it.

Addendum. It was lymphoma.

Rationalization

Br J Radiol. 2000 Jun;73(870):583-7. The characteristics and significance of thoracic lymphadenopathy in parapneumonic effusion and empyema. http://www.ncbi.nlm.nih.gov/pubmed/10911779

....

All In the Family?

How can I be so busy this week with so little to do? Every evening gone before I can sit at the Mac to write a case history. But my son was excellent as the King of Hearts in the Alice in Wonderland at the middle school.

The patient has the onset of fevers, nausea and a fever while on dialysis and is admitted to the hospital for possible early sepsis. She notes some mild abdominal pain and diarrhea, but the history fails to yield a reason for an infectious diarrhea—no dietary indiscretions or recent antibiotics. As if anyone needs unusual dietary consumption for an infectious diarrhea. As best I can tell, the world and everything we eat is covered with a thin layer of poo and, sometimes, GI pathogens.

It is why I only eat fried foods. With the advent of deep fried beer my last obstacle to pathogen-free dining has been removed.

However, a careful history reveals that a month ago at Thanksgiving, the meal was in part prepared by a family member being treated for *C. difficile* diarrhea. Although no one else who was at the meal is currently suffering from the Hershey squirts, I start to wonder if there is a link.

C. difficile has caused nosocomial and nursing home outbreaks, but I can find no information relating to *C. difficile* being spread person-to-person in households.

And what would the incubation period be from exposure to

C. difficile if the *C. difficile* is not due to antibiotics? Again not known, at least that I can find. Most studies suggest a 1 to 7 day time for colitis after antibiotics are started. Given that *C. difficile* has been found in most meats and fast food salads, given the time from the potential exposure, it may be an inadvertent dietary exposure (and are they all not inadvertent? Who wakes up in the morning and says, today I eat *C. difficile?*).

On the other hand, which is why I wash them frequently, *Clostridium* forms spores, so it could easily have potentially hid in her GI tract for a month.

And what is the infectious dose? Not known.

She is not on an acid suppressor, which is a risk for community-acquired and nosocomial *C. difficile*—which would also suggest that it is new consumption bacteria that is the proximate cause of many cases of *C. difficile*. I can't see how gastric acid would otherwise help prevent a colonic process. *C. difficile* without classic risk factors is probably more common that appreciated

Fifty-eight cases of CO-CDI were diagnosed among a total community population of 418,000, representing an estimated prevalence of CO-CDI of 1.29 per 10,000. All 58 cases were successfully contacted, representing a 100% response rate. Four cases were excluded from further analysis due to co-infection with Salmonella spp. and Campylobacter spp. Cases were more likely to be female, aged between 31 and 40 years, and present in the spring season (March–May), 2009. 46.3% (25/54) of cases had established risk factors for CDI, 20.4% (11/54) had non-established risk factors, 16.7% (9/54) had no risk factors and in the remaining 16.7% (9/54), available information was insufficient to classify by risk factor category.

I have a suspicion the epidemiology of *C. difficile* is a tad more complicated than suspected. The other source, besides food, could be the resident vermin, er, I mean dogs and cats, which can also carry *C. difficile*. Yet another reason to avoid pet 'therapy' in the hospital unless the animal is autoclaved first.

Rationalization

Use of Gastric Acid–Suppressive Agents and the Risk of Community-Acquired Clostridium difficile–Associated Disease. JAMA. http://jama.ama-assn.org/content/294/23/2989.abstract

J Infect Public Health. 2010;3(3):118-23. Epub 2010 Aug 23. Epidemiology of community-onset Clostridium difficile infection in a community in the South of England http://www.ncbi.nlm.nih.gov/pubmed/20869672

Clinical Infectious Diseases 2010;51:577–582. Clostridium difficile in Food and Domestic Animals: A New Foodborne Pathogen? http://www.journals.uchicago.edu/doi/full/10.1086/655692

My favorite dietary source for *C. difficile* is
- hamburger. 30%
- salads. 27%
- pork. 3%
- cat. The other other white meat. 33%
- dog. 0%
- Other Answers 7%
    Long pork

·····················

A Return To the Bad Old Days

DISEASES come and go. Sometimes for unknown reasons. Do you ever wonder what happened to the English Sweating Sickness? I do. There were six outbreaks between 1485 and 1551, it killed thousands, then disappeared never to be seen again. What was it? No one knows. Where did it come from and where did it go? Also unknown. Will it come back? I sure hope not. Would Axe deodorant help? Probably, if you believe the commercials.

Other diseases have almost vanished thanks to modern medicine, but, for a variety of social reasons, make an occasional reappearance.

The patient is a young West African who presents with a seizure. The CT scan of his brain shows four irregular lesions with edema, and the labs show a pancytopenia with a CD4 count of 40 cells per cubic millimeter. A count of less than 200 defines AIDS in an HIV-infected person. He denies HIV risks, but his HIV test is positive on the enzyme immunoassay (EIA) and the confirmatory Western blot is pending.

The rule with HIV-related CNS masses is: single lesion, toxoplasma serology negative means cancer, get a biopsy. Multiple lesions, toxoplasma negative: cancer, get a biopsy. Multiple lesions, toxoplasma positive: treat for toxoplasma. Single lesion, toxoplasma positive: treat and see if it gets better in 10 days or so.

His toxoplasma IgG antibody is greater than the upper limit of normal for the assay (1:2000 or so) so it is a safe bet it is toxoplasmosis.

CNS toxoplasmosis is reactivation disease in most HIV patients. They usually acquire it from not from cats, as is popularly thought, but from diet. The association depends on where you live, with some areas having more risks from diet than others. I still remember getting rare fowl in France. Still, to be safe autoclave the cat during pregnancy.

Turns out the patient has known that he has AIDS for at least five years, but told no one and did not seek care. It was due to a fear of being deported commingled with the opinion that HIV is a government plot against Africans. The latter is not an uncommon opinion in some communities, including large parts of Africa, and is a difficult worldview to change. Tuskegee and its many cousins makes it hard to defend a counterargument that unethical human experimentation is ludicrous and modern governments would not be involved with any such evil.

I hope he decides to take therapy this time around.

Addendum. He didn't. He vanished after discharge.

Rationalization

The English Sweating Sickness, 1485 to 1551. http://www.nejm.org/doi/pdf/10.1056/NEJM199702203360812

Epidemiol Infect. 2005 June; 133(3): 475–483. Risk factors for toxoplasmosis in pregnant women in Kent, United Kingdom. http://www.ncbi.nlm.nih.gov/pmc/articles/PMC2870271/

Three Thousand Words Plus a Few More

Let us start with the pictures.

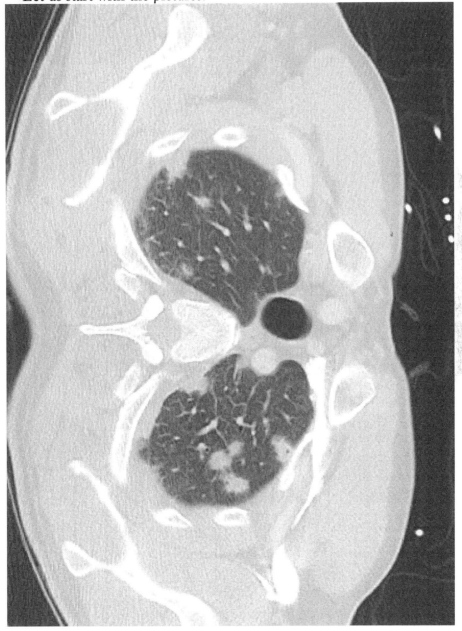

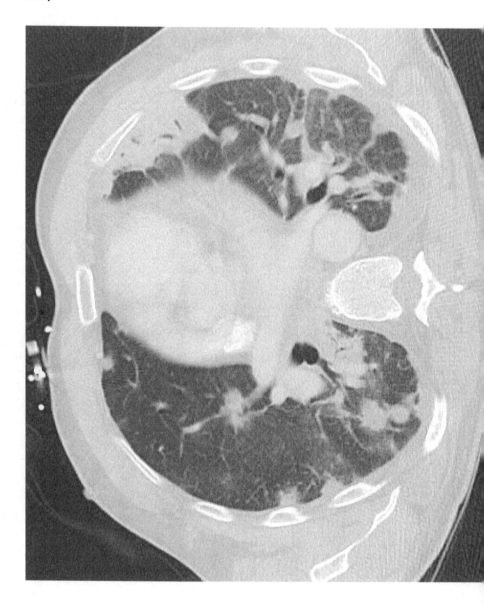

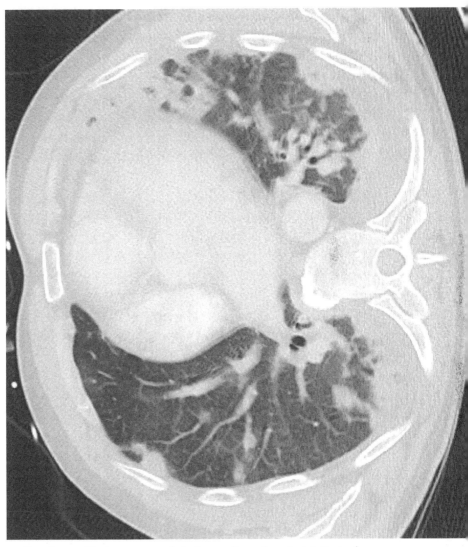

Look at all those round lesions. So what is it? It isn't tumor, although that was the initial worry.

Initially the patient is too ill to give a good history. He has no past medical history at all. Zip. He has nothing on exam. Zip. His labs have a leukocytosis but nothing else.

Transthoracic echocardiography (TTE) shows maybe, maybe not, a vegetation on the tricuspid valve. Not the best quality study. Endocarditis? *Staphylococcus* will do this, makes a patient acutely ill with lots of emboli, but usually the vegetation is not subtle and it is always nice to have a reason for endocarditis. He has zero risk factors; still, my practice is based on the fact that people get terrible infections for no reason at all.

Next day, the blood is growing gram positive cocci in chains and pairs. Could be streptococcus, could be pneumococcus.

Either way it's odd. Streptococcal endocarditis is more indolent, is unusual on the right side—and again, there's no reason for him to have it. No way am I having a fourth case of pneumococcal endocarditis.

Two days later the patient is better, able to give a history. It all started with a severe left-sided sore throat. No preceding trauma or dental work, his teeth are just fine.

Is this Lemierre's syndrome—post-anginal sepsis, aka septic thrombophlebitis of the internal jugular? Usually Lemierre's is due to bad teeth and *Fusobacterium*, but all these emboli would be more likely with Lemmiere's. Still, it is not typical for either endocarditis or Lemmiere's. To sort things out, a transesophageal echocardiogram is rock normal and his internal jugular is filled with clot. So Lemierre's it is.

The streptococcus? The lab calls it a viridans streptococcus, but when I call them to ask what the machine says, it's 90% likely *S. pluranimalium*. Oral strep are quantum bacteria, and the streptococcal wave function has to collapse into a probability of identification: *S. pluranimalium*. I wonder whether if I fire individual viridans streptococci through a single slit if they would form an interference pattern.

What is *S. pluranimalium*? I never heard of it, but there are three case reports of other viridans streptococci causing Lemierre's.

The new species S. pluranimalium was described by Devriese et al. The strains resembled S. acidominimus, and in fact some of the reference strains of S. acidominimus in culture collections were reidentified as S. pluranimalium. S. pluranimalium has been isolated from bovine mastitis; bovine vagina, cervix, and tonsils; and canary lung and lesions. No human isolates have been confirmed.

It is as true today as in 2002: there are no cases reported in humans by that name in PubMed, although it can cause endocarditis in chickens. Who knew chickens were heroin users? I know. A fowl pun.

The patient has no animal exposures and all streptococci die when faced with penicillin.

Rationalization

Clinical Microbiology Reviews, October 2002, p. 613-630, Vol. 15, No. 4. What Happened to the Streptococci: Overview of Taxonomic and Nomenclature Changes. http://cmr.asm.org/cgi/content/full/15/4/613

Avian Pathol. 2009 Apr;38(2):155-60. Association of Streptococcus pluranimalium with valvular endocarditis and septicaemia in adult broiler parents. http://www.ncbi.nlm.nih.gov/pubmed/19322715

Bad Bug, Bad Bug. Watcha Gonna Do, Watcha Gonna Do When I Come For You?

THERE are the occasional infections I can't cure with antibiotics alone. Today's patient is an 80-year-old female with underlying lung disease: recurrent hemoptysis from diffuse alveolar hemorrhage. She has had an extensive workup at multiple hospitals, with every known test and no diagnosis. Some sort of vasculitis, it is supposed, but no one has ever been able to put a name on it. It is treated with steroids. Her pulmonary compromise has led to a tracheostomy and her sputum always has a pan-susceptible *Burkholderia cepacia* complex. Why a complex?

B. cepacia is a genetically highly diverse class of bacteria, which is composed of several different species and discrete groups constituting the B. cepacia complex. Each group differs sufficiently from the others to constitute a species, and those that are phenotypically distinct have been assigned species designation. Those that cannot be differentiated phenotypically but are genetically distinct are defined as genomovars. As phenotypic differentiation among the genomovars has improved over the past decade, new species designa-

tion has been assigned as follows: genomovar II = B. multivorans, genomovar IV = B. stabilis, genomovar V = B. vietnamiensis, and genomovar VII = B. ambifaria. Genomovars I and III cannot be differentiated phenotypically, nor can B. multivorans and genomovar VI; these species must be distinguished by genetic methods. Bacteria from each of the genomovars have been recovered from patients with CF, but the predominant isolates in North America are from genomovar III and B. multivorans.

Yeah. I would call that complex.

She also has a prosthetic mitral valve and a dual chamber pacemaker. If you think this is sounding ominous, you are correct, Sir or Ma'am as the case may be.

She has acute respiratory decline and is intubated and placed on cefepime, a semi-synthetic cephalosporin antibiotic, and is initially stable in the ICU.

She does not quite get better and blood cultures, drawn due to fever on day three of antibiotics, are positive for *Burkholderia* after three days. More blood cultures are drawn and again are positive three days later in the face of cefepime. The pneumonia is better radiographically, although the patient is slowly sliding into multiorgan system failure.

I think either the valve or the pacer system is infected with the *Burkholderia*. No other source is found, such as a line infection. As I have harped on many times in the past, the *sine qua non* of an endovascular infection is sustained bacteremia, which she has.

Transthoracic echocardiography shows no pathology, but I did not expect it to. What to do is problematic. I can't treat the infection medically if it involves the endovascular material and the patient is not a surgical candidate; she can't even tolerate a transesophageal echo.

Burkholderia does cause the occasional prosthetic valve endocarditis, usually early, and one pacer pocket infection is reported. As a rule, this beast is hard to kill when it doesn't involve prosthetic material. *Burkholderia* is often a problem in cystic fibrosis patients, where it is resistant to most antibiotics.

In the end she was transitioned to comfort care.

Rationalization

J Antimicrob Chemother. 2009 Sep;64 Suppl 1:i29-36. Has the era of untreatable infections arrived? http://jac.oxfordjournals.org/content/64/suppl_1/i29.long

Fatal Burkholderia cepacia early prosthetic valve endocarditis: a very rare case and a review of the literature. J Heart Valve Dis. 2005 Mar;14(2):271-4. http://www.ncbi.nlm.nih.gov/pubmed/15792192

Epidemiology of Burkholderia cepacia Complex in Patients with Cystic Fibrosis, Canada. http://www.cdc.gov/ncidod/eid/vol-8no2/01-0163.htm

Int J Syst Bacteriol. 1997 Oct;47(4):1188-200. Occurrence of multiple genomovars of Burkholderia cepacia in cystic fibrosis patients and proposal of Burkholderia multivorans sp. nov. http://ijs.sgmjournals.org/cgi/reprint/47/4/1188

Bad Bug by Space Ghost. http://www.actionext.com/names_g/ghost_space_lyrics/bad_bug_zorak.html

Unlike Love

SEVERAL years ago I treated a patient with cryptococcal meningitis and fungemia. She is normal, no immunological defects that I could find. She did not tolerate amphotericin B and has been on fluconazole for two years now. When I first saw her, her serum cryptococcal antigen was > 1:2064. Two years later it is 1:64. She still has *Cryptococcus*.

In the bad old HIV days before HAART, you knew that *Cryptococcus* was not curable, and that patients would be on lifetime suppressive fluconazole. This is the first time I have seen chronic disease is a normal host. Or is she normal?

There is an interesting and growing literature on the increased and decreased risk of infection due to polymorphisms in the Toll-like receptors. Yeast are controlled, in part, by the Toll-like receptor 4 pathway, and perhaps she has a mutation in that wing of the immune system that has made it impossible for her to control the *Cryptococcus*. Such a defect has been described for *Candida*, but not yet for *Cryptococcus* but is only a matter of time. I presume that most patients with odd organisms have some variation in the immune system that predisposed them to infection. I look forward to the day when, Dr. McCoy-like, I can slop the patient's DNA into a machine and find the mutations in the immune system that predispose them to infections.

It could be that it is not the host, but the organism. She has *C. gattii* and it is harder to kill and more virulent than *C. neoformans*, but I would still bet on a host immunologic defect and I may never be able to clear the infection. I have a saying: Unlike love, herpes is forever. Now I have to add *Cryptococcus* to the list.

The other curious bit of information is the source of the patient's *Cryptococcus*. I had presumed bad luck, as we see the occasional sporadic case of *Cryptococcus* in the Northwest, and the organism is slowly drifting south from its primary focus in Vancouver Island. One of the environmental reservoirs for *Cryptococcus* is cedar and fir trees.

C. gattii was isolated from the following five native tree species: alder (n = 5), cedar (n = 1), Douglas fir (n = 16), grand fir (n = 1), and Garry oak (n = 2). There were no positive samples from eucalypts.

As you may remember, *C. neoformans* is found in eucalypts. And I would have though the plural was eucalyptuseseseses.

I was talking with the patient about her exposure history and knew she worked with animals, but what I did not glean from the history several years ago is that she works in a barn where the floor is bark dust from cedars and firs that are made from trees from British Columbia and that she is often in a very dusty environment. Now I wonder if that was the source of the infection.

Today is December 25 and I would like to wish all my readers a generic nondenominational seasonal greeting.

When my kids were young I told them Santa was not allowed on the roof, since reindeer carry *Giardia*, *Anaplasma phagocytophilum*, and *Echinococcus granulosus*, and that is why they did not get presents. They were disappointed, but seemed to understand. It was important they develop an early fear of contagion.

Rationalization

Med Mycol. 2004 Dec;42(6):485-98. Toll-like receptors as key mediators in innate antifungal immunity. http://www.ncbi.nlm.nih.gov/pubmed/15682636

Eur Cytokine Netw. 2006 Mar;17(1):29-34. Toll-like receptor 4 Asp299Gly/Thr399Ile polymorphisms are a risk factor for Candida bloodstream infection. http://www.ncbi.nlm.nih.gov/pubmed/16613760

A rare genotype of Cryptococcus gattii caused the cryptococcosis outbreak on Vancouver Island (British Columbia, Canada). PNAS December 7, 2004 vol. 101 no. 49 17258-17263. http://www.pnas.org/content/101/49/17258.full

....

Not Quite an Explanation

THE patient is normal. Really normal. No risks for anything, living the quiet life of a student. He then has a week of fevers that were ascribed to asthma/ pneumonia due to a cough. He was treated with a course of doxycycline, and then, because of ongoing shortness of breath, he received a course of prednisone. While on the steroids he developed weakness in the left foot and had a seizure.

In the emergency room, everything was normal: physical exam, complete blood count, urinalysis, chest x-ray and, eventually, blood cultures. The CT and MRI of the brain showed 4 marble-sized irregular lesions with a lot of surrounding edema.

What are they? Tumor? Maybe. Cysticercosis, aka pork tapeworm? Could be. The patient was in South America six months ago, but they are not the nice round balls of fluid with a worm in them that you see with the typical cysticercosis. Bacterial? No reason. No shunt or IV drug use or endocarditis or anything.

So, which some trepidation, off to brain biopsy.

They were pockets of pus and grew *Staphylococcus intermedius* and *Enterococcus*.

Now where did those come from?

Brain abscesses occur either due to direct extension from a source in the head, usually sinusitis, or hematogenous spread, by way of the bloodstream. He has no reason for either, and the *Enterococcus* suggest a colonic source. And there is a paucity of reports of enterococcus causing brain abscess, so that organism makes this even odder.

The microbiology of brain abscess is more complicated than simple cultures would suggest. Using 16S ribosomal sequencing, it was recently discovered that brain abscess are richer in bacteria than expected.

The obtained cultures identified significantly fewer types of bacteria (22 strains) than did molecular testing (72 strains; P = .017, by analysis of variance test). We found that a patient could exhibit as many as 16 different bacterial species in a single abscess. The obtained cultures identified 14 different species already known to cause cerebral abscess. Single sequencing performed poorly, whereas multiple sequencing identified 49 species, of which 27 had not been previously reported in brain abscess investigations and 15 were completely unknown. Interestingly, we observed 2 patients who harbored Mycoplasma hominis (an emerging pathogen in this situation) and 3 patients who harbored Mycoplasma faucium, which, to our knowledge, has never been reported in literature.

So, looking for a reason, he had what some call the Pan Scan: CT of chest, abdomen and pelvis, which found an inflammatory mass next to the esophagus that was, on biopsy, an infection.

The presumption is this a complication of an esophageal perforation. What goes against this is he remembers no specific dietary trauma that could have lead to a hole in the esophagus.

Here are the two "best" perforations I have seen in my time ("best" as in "most curious"). One was a bread clip, the square pieces of plastic used on bread bags, that eroded through the large bowel. How the clip could be inadvertently eaten, ate, ated, consumed, I never discovered. Years ago my intern was eating breakfast post-call and he complained that the bran muffin was chewier than usual; it turned out he was eating the paper the muffin was baked in.

The other, and more commonly reported, is the tortilla chip. Unchewed, they are like swallowing a ninja star. I had a patient who, while a wee bit inebriated, did not chew his tortilla chip and it ripped him a new one in his esophagus, with a resultant complicated mediastinal abscess.

So was the cough and the shortness of breath due to the esophageal leak and the steroids turned a local infection into a disseminated one? No idea. It is one of those cases that is frustratingly close to a unifying answer, but not quite there.

And chew your food, especially the sharp food.

Rationalization

Clin Infect Dis. 2009 May 1;48(9):1169-78. The expansion of the microbiological spectrum of brain abscesses with use of multiple 16S ribosomal DNA sequencing. http://cid.oxfordjournals.org/content/48/9/1169.full

N Engl J Med. 1990 May 10;322(19):1399-400. Esophageal tear caused by a tortilla chip. http://www.ncbi.nlm.nih.gov/pubmed/2325744

AJR Am J Roentgenol. 1983 Mar;140(3):503-4. Food laceration of the esophagus: the taco tear. http://www.ncbi.nlm.nih.gov/pubmed/6600542

POLL RESULTS
- The most dangerous thing to swallow is
- a bread clip. 4%
- a taco shell. 15%
- a sword. 4%
- a declaration of undying love after a six pack. 35%
- a campaign promise. 37%
- Other Answers 4%
- 1   inflammatory health propaganda
- 2   a sewing needle

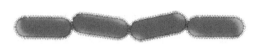

Billed As One Thing, Turns Out To Be Another.

THE patient is a middle-aged female who has an issue with her hip. It was replaced three years and kept dislocating, so she had two revisions over a year, then a new hip. Initially the second joint was fine, then she developed a tender ball over the incision that "squirted across the room when it ruptured." While this volcanic boil was growing she had no fevers or chills. She was told it was an MRSA infection and treated with a course of vancomycin with no effect. It continued to drain and she was transferred to my institution for hip removal and was billed as a chronic MRSA hip infection.

Past medical history includes diabetes, multiple joint replacements, and a distant MRSA infection of a back surgical wound a decade ago.

The exam is negative as are the screening labs.

The cultures from the outside hospital from earlier in the year did not grow MRSA; they had pus but no growth. Still, the vancomycin was a reasonable choice to treat a culture-negative hip infection, since coagulase negative staphylococci are the most likely uncultured organism.

She goes off to have her hip explanted and everything grows *Candida albicans*. Not the organism I would have predicted.

The surgeon said it did not look like a typical bacterial infection, but there was a lot of grungy tissue. This is the Great Pacific Northwest, so I assume it meant he found torn jeans and a flannel shirt in the hip.

Was *Candida* there before? Maybe. *Candida* can be indolent and perhaps the outside lab didn't hold the cultures long enough. Or maybe the MRSA was cured and this is a secondary infection. There is no way to know for sure.

Candida infections in prosthetic joints are not that common with 30 references on a PubMed search, maybe 12 infections in the hip.

"We identified 7 patients, 4 with knee and 3 with hip prosthetic infections. The most frequent fungal agent was Candida albicans (4 cases), followed by Candida parapsilosis (2 cases) and Candida guillermondii (1 case). All the patients received antifungal treatment for a prolonged period. Five patients had their prosthesis removed and 3 had reimplantation, 1 patient was treated with debridement and prosthetic retention, and the last patient refused surgery. The mean follow-up time was 2.5 y. At the last evaluation, 3 patients were considered as cured, 3 patients presented a secondary bacterial infection leading to amputation for 2 of them, and 1 patient died from heart failure"

Best treatment? No good data, but now that the hip has been explanted I have opted for relatively high dose fluconazole. The literature consists of cases and case series, and the plural of anecdote is anecdotes, not data.

There are cases cured with monotherapy as well as a variety of combination therapies:

"Candida prosthetic joint infection is a rare clinical entity, and only 12 cases of Candida albicans prosthetic hip infection have been described. Although surgery combined with a long period of antifungal medication is the usual treatment for fungal prosthetic joint infections, monotherapy with antifungal agents has only very rarely been used as a therapeutic option, especially in debilitated and elderly patients. We report herein the second case, to our knowledge, of C. albicans prosthetic hip arthritis successfully treated with fluconazole monotherapy and review the literature on the pathogenesis, clinical manifestations and management of these infections. Further studies on the use of fluconazole in the management of fungal prosthetic infections are needed."

The only problem with that conclusion is that you need a large number of fungal prosthetic hip infections for study, and that is probably not forthcoming any time soon. It is akin to my least favorite conclusion in a paper, where a once-in-a- millennium infection is presented and the authors suggest that all doctors need to consider the odd diagnosis in the future. I bet they never pass up an opportunity to mention the once-in-a-lifetime-of-the-universe infection at every opportunity.

Rationalization

Scand J Infect Dis. 2010 Dec;42(11-12):890-5. Epub 2010 Jul 7.

Candida prosthetic infections: case series and literature review. http://www.ncbi.nlm.nih.gov/pubmed/20608769

Scand J Infect Dis. 2010;42(1):12-21. Candida albicans prosthetic hip infection in elderly patients: is fluconazole monotherapy an option? http://www.ncbi.nlm.nih.gov/pubmed/20055725

What To Do Now?

PROBLEMS without a good answer. That defines my life and this book.

A couple of years ago I treated a patient with chronic coccidioidomycosis pneumonia.

Over a year he slowly improved, both radiographically and by the serum complement fixation assay, which measures antibodies to the fungus. He is/was a diabetic, but did not have meningitis.

He had reasonably severe pneumonia, a very high coccidioidomycosis complement fixation titer, and a low threshold for renal toxicity from amphotericin. His kidneys shut down after a few doses of lipid amphotericin, and he did not tolerate relatively high dose fluconazole, but toughed it out until the point where I thought we had a "cure." Quotes around a word. Like "fresh" fish, quotes tend to cast doubt on the truthiness of the word they surround.

Two years after finishing the fluconazole the patient has a growth on his arm that is thought to be a cyst. Anyone reading this think it's going to be a cyst? Of course not. This is an ID story. The cyst was removed and, there at the center, like the middle of an infectious tootsie roll pop, is coccidioidomycosis. For those who like numbers, it takes as few as 50 and as many as 1500 licks to get to the center of a tootsie roll pop, depending on the length of lick, the amount of saliva on the tongue and other factors.

Now what? Amphotericin? That was a disaster last time. Back on fluconazole? One definition of insanity is repeating a process and seeing if you have a different outcome.

The literature suggests that 800 mg of posaconazole is a good choice for refractory cocci with a good outcome:

"Patients were refractory to previous therapy (including ampho-tericin B with or without an azole) for a median duration of 306 days. At the end of treatment (posaconazole treatment duration, 34 to 365 days), therapy for 11 of 15 patients (73%) was consid-ered to be successful by the DRC. Four responses were complete and seven were partial; these included five patients with pulmonary sites and six patients with disseminated sites. In responders, im-provement was seen within months of the initiation of therapy. Five patients received therapy for >or= 12 months. The side effects were minimal."

Downside? At that dose it is going to cost an arm, a leg and the firstborn male child. Wholesale, and who pays wholesale, about 740 bucks every 5 days. A three hundred day course? 44,000 dol-lars. And that's wholesale. That's a good chunk of change, I had better get really good pizza at the next conference. But I do not see that the patient has any better alternatives.

Rationalization

Chest. 2007 Sep;132(3):952-8. Epub 2007 Jun 15. Posaconazole ther-apy for chronic refractory coccidioidomycosis. http://www.ncbi.nlm.nih.gov/pubmed/17573510

Clin Infect Dis. 2005 Jun 15;40(12):1770-6. Epub 2005 May 13. Re-fractory coccidioidomycosis treated with posaconazole. http://www.ncbi.nlm.nih.gov/pubmed/15909265

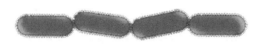

Who Needs The Influenza Vaccine? Guess My Answer

THIS is a break from the usual short romp through pus that characterizes this book. .

Do Healthy Adults Really Need a Flu Shot?

The evidence for influenza vaccination is like the evidence for evolution: there are multiple lines of evidence that demonstrate the multiple benefits of influenza vaccination.

The best way to get long-lasting immunity against a given strain of influenza is to get infected. If you survive the infection and its potential complications, you will have lifelong immunity against that strain of flu. Lifelong immunity is what allowed the elderly to have decreased mortality during the H1N1 pandemic: they were resistant to the virus, having had flu with the strain of H1N1 that circulated until the middle of last century.

The problem with using illness to develop immunity is the morbidity and mortality that result from contagion. Influenza, depending of the year and the circulating strains, can cause significant illness and death. Vaccination would be a better option; an ounce of prevention and all that.

What can be said about the flu vaccine? Vaccination has multiple potential effects. The effects of vaccination are more than a simple get the vaccine, don't get influenza.

"A single measure of vaccine efficacy fails to capture the multidimensional protective effect of vaccination. Individual vaccination can prevent or reduce a number of outcomes, including laboratory-confirmed infection, symptomatic illness given infection, infectivity of infected individuals, or a combination of these."

The vaccine elicits antibody to the strains found in the vaccine, and usually a high titer of antibody is protective.

One of the reasons that the vaccine is not as good at eliciting an immune response as getting an infection is that 10 days of unrestrained viral replication during active influenza presents the body with far more antigens in kind and quantity to respond to. The immune response to the vaccine is not as robust as it is to a natural infection, and part of the reason why the flu vaccine is not 100% efficacious.

In challenge trials, the vaccine is moderately efficacious in preventing flu.

Challenge trials are the best-case scenario. You have a population that has a known response to the vaccine, gets a matched influenza strain up the nose at a known time and the vaccine prevents influenza. Not 100% of the time. And challenge studies are not the real world, but a good proof of concept.

"Protection rate against artificial challenge with influenza A was 96% when vaccine and challenge viruses were homotypic. When the vaccine strain and challenges virus were heterotypic, protection ranged from 70-100%. Protection rate from infection during a homotypic epidemic was, retrospectively, 95%; while 50-87% protection from influenza illness was achieved during a heterotypic epidemic. In all instances, vaccinees experienced mild, mostly afebrile upper respiratory symptoms, unlike controls who had moderate to severe symptoms, often with fever. Infecting virus was shed more often by unvaccinated controls."

Even if you do not prevent flu with the vaccine, those who get the vaccine are less ill, shed less virus, and are less likely to spread disease. No small thing, decreasing the spread of contagious diseases.

The biggest issue with the vaccine each year is predicting the strains to go in the vaccine months before the actual strains circulate. Sometimes they pick the strains in the vaccine with a good antigenic match to the circulating strains, and sometimes not so well, which leads to variability of vaccine efficacy in the real world.

Still, there is maybe the not-so-unexpected side effect that a mismatched strain this year may be protective against future strains of flu. Those who had swine flu vaccination in 1976 had some immunity against the 2009 strain. Flu vaccine efficacy is more than absolute prevention, and having some cross immunity from prior vaccinations could lead to a milder case of influenza in the future.

Vaccination of populations leads to decreases in disease and decreased deaths.

A problem with all the vaccine trials and influenza vaccination in general is we have never had vaccination rates that reach the 90-95% rates required for herd immunity to kick in and prevent influenza from spreading. So everyone who gets the vaccine, which is can be only modestly effective some years, is thrown into the general cesspool of circulating influenza to either get the flu or be in a susceptible population to ensure continued spread of the disease.

The greater the uptake of influenza vaccination in a population, the less the death during flu season. The most compelling population data comes from Ontario, Canada, where they have had a ongoing attempt to maximize vaccination of the whole population against influenza. The other provinces did not see fit to try and vaccinate everyone, continuing with targeted influenza vaccination.

This represents an interesting natural experiment. If the effects of the influenza vaccine are less in preventing disease but more in decreasing secondary endpoints like death, hospitalizations, or antibiotic usage, it may show up in population studies. There are numerous issues with this kind of study, but are "appropriate for assessing the public health impact of a population-wide intervention."

During the period, Ontario experienced greater uptake of vaccine than any other Province:

"Between the pre-UIIP 1996–1997 estimate to the mean post-UIIP vaccination rate, influenza vaccination rates for the household population aged ≥12 y increased 20 percentage points (18%–38%) for Ontario, compared to 11 percentage points (13%–24%) for other provinces (p < 0.001) (Table 2). For those <65 y, the

vaccination rate increases were greater in Ontario than in other provinces, while for those ≥75 y, the increase was smaller in Ontario. For all age groups, Ontario always achieved higher vaccination rates than other provinces."

And the results of all that vaccination:

"After UIIP introduction, influenza-associated mortality for the overall population decreased 74% in Ontario (RR = 0.26, 95% confidence interval [CI], 0.20–0.34) compared to 57% in other provinces (RR = 0.43, 95% CI, 0.37–0.50) (ratio of RRs = 0.61, p = 0.002) (Table 3). In age-specific analyses, larger mortality decreases in Ontario were found to be statistically significant only in those ≥85 y."

Not bad.

"Overall, influenza-associated health care use decreased more in Ontario than other provinces for hospitalizations (RR = 0.25 versus 0.44, ratio of RRs = 0.58, p < 0.001), ED use (RR = 0.31 versus 0.70, ratio of RRs = 0.45, p < 0.001), and doctors' office visits (RR = 0.21 versus 0.53, ratio of RRs = 0.41, p < 0.001). In age-specific analyses, greater decreases were consistently observed in Ontario than other provinces for age groups <65 y. For seniors, greater decreases were observed in Ontario than other provinces for hospitalizations among those aged 65–84 y and for ED use among those 65–74 y."

Increasing vaccination rates in children decreases influenza in the community.

"Considerable evidence indicates that herd immunity is operative in the control of influenza as well. In Tecumseh, Michigan, 85% of 3159 schoolchildren were given TIV over 4 days and compared to a similar population in the neighboring community of Adrian, where vaccine was not administered. Three times more influenza-like illness occurred among people of all ages in Adrian than in Tecumseh, demonstrating that immunizing school children in a community significantly protects the population at large in that community."

Influenza vaccination of pregnant women, one of the groups at high risk for death from flu, also decreases flu and hospitalization in their newborns.

Flu vaccine may, in part, prevent death from vascular events. There are two ongoing themes in the ID literature that have yet to overlap. One is people who get severe infections that require hospitalization not only have increased short term mortality, but long term mortality as well. Why they die is not as well worked out, but in those who die after pneumonia have increased inflammatory markers at discharge.

The other theme is that inflammation is a pro-thombotic state and patients with acute infections are more likely to have strokes, heart attacks and pulmonary embolisms, and that risk of vascular events can be elevated for up to a year. Even an aggressive tooth cleaning increases the risk for a vascular event.

The rate of vascular events significantly increased in the first 4 weeks after invasive dental treatment (incidence ratio, 1.50 [95% CI, 1.09 to 2.06]) and gradually returned to the baseline rate within 6 months.

Infection leads to inflammation leads to clot leads to vascular events. If you could stop that cascade, say with a vaccine, you could conceivably decrease the number of deaths from vascular events. And so it does with a combination of the flu and pneumococcal vaccine.

"Of the 36,636 subjects recruited, 7292 received both PPV and TIV, 2076 received TIV vaccine alone, 1875 received PPV alone, and 25,393 were unvaccinated, with a duration of follow‚Äêup of 45,834 person‚Äêyears. Baseline characteristics were well matched between the groups, except that there were fewer male patients in the PPV and TIV group and fewer cases of comorbid chronic obstructive pulmonary disease among unvaccinated persons. At week 64 from commencement of the study, dual‚Äêvaccinees experienced fewer deaths (hazard ratio [HR], 0.65; 95% confidence interval [CI], 0.55‚Äì0.77]; P<.001) and fewer cases of pneumonia (HR, 0.57; 95% CI, 0.51‚Äì0.64; P<.001), ischemic stroke

(HR, 0.67; 95% CI, 0.54‚Äì0.83; P<.001), and acute myocardial infarction (HR, 0.52; 95% CI, 0.38‚Äì0.71; P<.001), compared with unvaccinated subjects. Dual vaccination resulted in fewer coronary (HR, 0.59; 95% CI, 0.44‚Äì0.79; P<.001) and intensive care admissions (HR, 0.45; 95% CI, 0.22‚Äì0.94; P=.03), compared with among unvaccinated subjects."

Note: the beneficial effects occurred up to 64 weeks after receiving the vaccines; influenza vaccine could conceivably protect from death outside of flu season because vaccination prevents the sustained detrimental inflammatory effect of infections.

The result does not hold true in every study, but the data suggests that the beneficial effects of preventing influenza are wide-ranging and not limited to avoiding an acute viral pneumonia. The effects of both influenza and the vaccine are more complicated than a simple flu vaccination prevents flu.

For those who worry about the H1N1 vaccine, a good match in the right population leads to excellent and safe protection against the flu:

"Through hospital-based active surveillance, 362 cases of incident neurologic diseases were identified within 10 weeks after the mass vaccination, including 27 cases of the Guillain-Barré syndrome. None of the neurologic conditions occurred among vaccine recipients. From 245 schools, 25,037 students participated in the mass vaccination and 244,091 did not. During the period from October 9 through November 15, 2009, the incidence of confirmed cases of 2009 H1N1 virus infection per 100,000 students was 35.9 (9 of 25,037) among vaccinated students and 281.4 (687 of 244,091) among unvaccinated students. Thus, the estimated vaccine effectiveness was 87.3% (95% confidence interval, 75.4 to 93.4)."

Please note: all the Guillain-Barré Syndrome was in the unvaccinated people.

These are some of the many studies that demonstrate that the effectiveness of the flu vaccine is multifactorial. There are over 16,000 references on PubMed if you search for "influenza vaccine." If you are bored, spend a day reading them, then tell me the flu vaccine doesn't work.

Which leads us to the Cochrane review. The Cochrane folks only review randomized, controlled trials and perform a systematic review/meta-analysis on the results. Their approach is narrow and they are fairly rigorous about applying their techniques, even to the point of ignoring reality. For example, they did a review on oscillococcinum, a flu "remedy."

If you are unaware of what is in oscillococcinum, it is prepared as follows.

> "Into a one litre bottle, a mixture of pancreatic juice and glucose is poured. Next a Canard de Barbarie (a duck) is decapitated and 35 grams of its liver and 15 grams of its heart are put into the bottle. Why liver? Doctor Roy writes: "The Ancients considered the liver as the seat of suffering, even more important than the heart, which is a very profound insight, because it is on the level of the liver that the pathological modifications of the blood happen, and also there the quality of the energy of our heart muscle changes in a durable manner."

After 40 days in the sterile bottle, liver and heart autolyse (disintegrate) into a kind of goo, which is then "potentized" with the Korsakov method where the glass containing the remedy is shaken and then just emptied and refilled with fresh water.

So you are washing out your stemware. How many times would you fill and swirl the glass with water before you considered the glass clean of wine and soap. Two times? Three? To make oscillococcinum they fill, shake, empty, and add fresh water to the bottle 200 times. A drop of the last dilution is placed on sugar pills.

By the time they are done, the duck goo can be found at one part duck goo in 100^{200} water molecules, which is damn impressive since there are only about 10^{80} $(+/- 3)$ total atoms in the entire observable universe. Anyone who thinks that oscillococcinum has any potential to treat influenza, well, we live in different universes. For reasons I cannot discover, the Cochrane review on homeopathy was withdrawn. Embarrassment would be my guess.

The Cochrane folks put out an update of their systematic review for the effectiveness of influenza. And their conclusions? It is not the greatest vaccine but effective.

"In the relatively uncommon circumstance of vaccine matching the viral circulating strain and high circulation, 4% of unvaccinated people versus 1% of vaccinated people developed influenza symptoms (risk difference (RD) 3%, 95% confidence interval (CI) 2% to 5%). The corresponding figures for poor vaccine matching were 2% and 1% (RD 1, 95% CI 0% to 3%). These differences were not likely to be due to chance. Vaccination had a modest effect on time off work and had no effect on hospital admissions or complication rates. Inactivated vaccines caused local harms and an estimated 1.6 additional cases of Guillain-Barré Syndrome per million vaccinations. The harms evidence base is limited.

AUTHORS' CONCLUSIONS: Influenza vaccines have a modest effect in reducing influenza symptoms and working days lost."

You get the feeling it pains them to admit the flu vaccine has efficacy, what with the caveat "In the relatively uncommon circumstance of vaccine matching the viral circulating strain and high circulation" and the choice of "modest" in the conclusion. And then, the weirdness in the abstract:

'WARNING: This review includes 15 out of 36 trials funded by industry (four had no funding declaration). An earlier systematic review of 274 influenza vaccine studies published up to 2007 found industry funded studies were published in more prestigious journals and cited more than other studies independently from methodological quality and size. Studies funded from public sources were significantly less likely to report conclusions favorable to the vaccines. The review showed that reliable evidence on influenza vaccines is thin but there is evidence of widespread manipulation of conclusions and spurious notoriety of the studies. The content and conclusions of this review should be interpreted in light of this finding."

Fine. Who pays for the study can subtly bias the outcomes. I have written about that before. It does not necessarily discredit a study, but you do have to read and interpret the studies carefully and take the conclusions with a bit of salt substitute.

That is where, I thought, a meta-analysis comes in. Someone like the Cochrane group reviews the data with no concern about the impact or quality of the journal or notoriety of the references. The Cochrane reviews, I thought, looked at the numbers unbiased by the spin in the conclusions or where the study was published. They let the studies survive or fall based on their quality.

I can only think of two reasons why this warning was published.

1) The authors do not like the conclusions from the data, and are undermining the result, spinning the abstract to try and sway the message casual readers will take away from the review. It always amazes me how often people parrot the spin in a paper, and papers have spin, with no independent thought.

or

2) The authors are saying they are biased by the conclusions in the papers and the notoriety of some studies and as a result their analysis of the data is not to be trusted. In other words, the Cochrane reviewers are incredulous rubes who just fell off the turnip truck and were sold a bill of goods by those vaccinating city slickers with their manipulated conclusions and spurious notoriety. So do not trust the Cochrane reviewers, they say so themselves.

Sad either way.

The discussion is odd, going beyond spin and wandering into petulant rants about past slights, with the authors saying that everyone misuses their meta-analysis and ignores the data.

"Both generalizations are not supported by any evidence and seem to originate from the desire to use our review to support decisions already taken. The misquotes appear to be based on both the abstract and Plain language summary (which is what you would expect from a superficial reading of the review by people with a specific agenda)."

They also use significant column inches to demonstrate just

how the ACIP misquoted them.

and

"The CDC authors clearly do not weight interpretation by quality of the evidence, but quote anything that supports their theory."

What a weird, petulant little potshot at the CDC. It could be that the CDC looks at multiple lines of evidence in concluding that the flu vaccine is a worthwhile medical intervention, not just the randomized clinical trials. Oh, I'm sorry, the Cochrane review has a monopoly on the truth and how complex clinical trials should be interpreted. My bad. We are not worthy, we are not worthy. Sorry the CDC does not defer to your omniscient truthiness.

"It used to be, everyone was entitled to their own opinion, but not their own facts. But that's not the case anymore. Facts matter not at all. Perception is everything. It's certainty... Truthiness is 'What I say is right, and [nothing] anyone else says could possibly be true.' It's not only that I feel it to be true, but that I feel it to be true. There's not only an emotional quality, but there's a selfish quality."

I could see a snitty statement like that maybe in an editorial, definitely in a popular text (but not this one, no way), but in the text of a major review? It makes me wonder if the Cochrane reviews have any editorial oversight for their content. If they do, then their editors have some splainin' to do as to how a major evidence based review could devolve to 'Mommy, mommy, I don't like the way the CDC is playing with my ball and they are calling me names. Make them stoooopppp.'

Sorry, dudes. Anyone group that evaluates oscillococcinum as if were based in reality is in no position to whine about quality when you participate in tooth fairy science. If you evaluate the flu vaccine using ALL the lines of evidence and look at ALL the potential benefits, it is not an unreasonable medical intervention.

It is probably projection on my part, but I find the Cochrane reviews on influenza vaccination to be biased against the flu vaccine in a subtle way that I do not see in the other reviews. The oscillococcinum review, while fundamentally stupid given the nature of the intervention, brainlessly followed the data, even though there was no plausibility for the intervention. They didn't try to spin the data.

The choice of adjectives used by the authors seem designed to cast doubt on vaccine efficacy. Now I am a vaccine proponent, and I could very well be reading into the text something that is not there. For an example, the plain language summary says

"Inactivated influenza vaccines decrease the risk of symptoms of influenza and time off work, but their effects are minimal, especially if the vaccines and the circulating viruses are mismatched."

Minimal: of a minimum amount, quantity, or degree; Their analysis says

"In the relatively uncommon circumstance of vaccine matching the viral circulating strain and high circulation, 4% of unvaccinated people versus 1% of vaccinated people developed influenza symptoms."

In a country the size of the US, that is the difference between 12 million and 3 million getting flu if everyone were vaccinated (yes, I know, all 300,000,000 Americans are not healthy adults). Worst case, it would be 6 million vs. 3 million. Still, across the whole population of the country, that would not be a minimal effect.

Or the number needed to treat:

"The combined results of these trials showed that under ideal conditions (vaccine completely matching circulating viral configuration) 33 healthy adults need to be vaccinated to avoid one set of influenza symptoms."

And that does not include all the potential downstream effects of vaccination by preventing a case and its complications and spread. It is like seatbelts and airbags. They do not prevent all mortality and morbidity in an accident, but I would prefer both as I drive around the city.

Flu vaccine seems good intervention, a reasonable bang for

the buck. I would say it is often a moderately effective vaccine, sometimes, as in the case of H1N1, an excellent vaccine, with widespread health benefits beyond the prevention of acute influenza. The cost effectiveness of flu vaccination is debatable and is ultimately a value judgment. In medicine they try and calculate the quality-adjusted life-year of an intervention to see if it is worth it to society.

It is form of evaluation that makes my brain hurt, and I lack the knowledge to do much except to take them at face value. The outcome of cost-effectiveness evaluations depends on the assumptions made. For the elderly, you get conclusions like this:

"Vaccination was cost saving, i.e., it both reduced medical expenses and improved health, for all age groups and geographic areas analyzed in the base case. For people aged 65 years and older, vaccination saved $8.27 and gained 1.21 quality-adjusted days of life per person vaccinated. Vaccination of the 23 million elderly people unvaccinated in 1993 would have gained about 78 000 years of healthy life and saved $194 million. In univariate sensitivity analysis, the results remained cost saving except for doubling vaccination costs, including future medical costs of survivors, and lowering vaccination effectiveness. With assumptions most unfavorable to vaccination, cost per quality-adjusted life-year ranged from $35,822 for ages 65 to 74 years to $598,487 for ages 85 years and older."

In the US a cost per quality-adjusted life-year of around $50,000 is considered acceptable for an intervention.

It appears to me that the authors of the Cochrane reviews think flu vaccination is not a worthwhile public health intervention, which is fine, but quit being a weasel and hiding behind words like minimal and complaining that people misuse your reviews for their own ends. The get close to admitting this in the discussion:

"Given the limited availability of resources for mass immunization, the use of influenza vaccines should be primarily directed where there is clear evidence of benefit."

If I waited for clear evidence in medicine I would treat no one. But, to quote Donald Rumsfeld, I have to fight the wars with the weapons I have. However, the preponderance of data from basic principles to epidemiology to clinical trials leads me to conclude that the flu vaccine is moderately effective and cost effective. Someday, I hope, they will develop the universal flu vaccine and then, with universal vaccination, we will go all smallpox vaccination on influenza.

The Cochrane reviewers give the appearance of being thin-skinned, petulant, whiny, babies with a bias against flu vaccination. BTW. It is not an *ad hominem* since I do not think the review is wrong or flawed because they are crybabies. The substance is fine, the tone of the spin is whiny crybaby. Boo frigity hoo. Got an issue? Here's a tissue.

Either way, the confidence I have in the Cochrane reviews, at least as far as influenza vaccine goes, is now at an all time low.

So who should get the flu vaccine? Everyone.

Is it a perfect vaccine? Nope.

Does it prevent flu and many complications of flu? Yep.

Is it cost effective? Worth the effort? My opinion is yes, but that is a judgment call.

If you are a young healthy adult, do you want to decrease you chances of flu? Or do you hate your elderly grandparents and want an untraceable way to kill them off so you can inherit their beachfront property? Do not get the flu vaccine and visit them when you start to get a fever and a cough.

Should you be wary of the spin the Cochrane reviews? You betcha.

Do Healthy Adults Really Need a Flu Shot?

Damn right they do.

Cherry Picked Rationalizations

Clin Infect Dis. 2010 Jun 1;50(11):1487-92. Recipients of vaccine against the 1976 "swine flu" have enhanced neutralization responses to the 2009 novel H1N1 influenza virus. http://www.ncbi.nlm.nih.gov/pubmed/20415539

Eur Respir J. 2010 Nov 11. Inflammatory response predict long-term mortality risk in community-acquired pneumonia.

http://www.ncbi.nlm.nih.gov/pubmed/21071473

Ann Intern Med. 2010 Oct 19;153(8):499-506. Invasive dental treatment and risk for vascular events: a self-controlled case series. http://www.ncbi.nlm.nih.gov/pubmed/20956706

Clin Infect Dis. 2010 Nov 1;51(9):1007-16. Prevention of acute myocardial infarction and stroke among elderly persons by dual pneumococcal and influenza vaccination: a prospective cohort study. http://www.ncbi.nlm.nih.gov/pubmed/20887208

N Engl J Med. 2010 Dec 16;363(25):2416-23. Safety and effectiveness of a 2009 H1N1 vaccine in Beijing. http://www.ncbi.nlm.nih.gov/pubmed/21158658

Influenza vaccine given to pregnant women reduces hospitalization due to influenza in their infants. Benowitz I, Esposito DB, Gracey KD, Shapiro ED, Vázquez M. Clin Infect Dis. 2010 Dec 15;51(12):1355-61. Epub 2010 Nov 8.

http://www.ncbi.nlm.nih.gov/pubmed/21058908

The True Story of Oscillococcinum. http://www.homeowatch.org/history/oscillo.html

Estimating Influenza Vaccine Efficacy From Challenge and Community-based Study Data Oxford JournalsMedicineAmerican Journal of Epidemiology Volume168, Issue12Pp. 1343-1352.

http://aje.oxfordjournals.org/content/168/12/1343.full

Dev Biol Stand. 1977 Jun 1-3;39:149-54. Challenge versus natural infection as an index or protection after influenza immunization. http://www.ncbi.nlm.nih.gov/pubmed/342306

PLoS Med. 2008 Oct 28;5(10):e211. The effect of universal influenza immunization on mortality and health care use. http://www.ncbi.nlm.nih.gov/pubmed/18959473

Bull World Health Organ. 1969;41(3):537-42. Effect of vaccination of a school-age population upon the course of an A2-Hong Kong influenza epidemic.

http://www.ncbi.nlm.nih.gov/pubmed/5309469

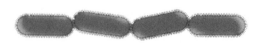

Empiricism?

I F I have a flaw as a clinician (and, depending on who you ask, I may or may not have many), it is that I tend to focus more on diagnosis than treatment, and sometimes you need to treat before you get all the diagnostic data back. It doesn't matter the site or the organism, if appropriate antibiotic therapy is delayed in the ICU, mortality goes up every hour and every day. So sometime you have to pull the trigger before you know for sure what you are aiming at. Be glad you do not hunt with me.

The patient is a young diabetic, in renal failure and on dialysis, with paraparesis. Initially she has *C. difficile* and perhaps a line infection, but despite appropriate therapy she only gets worse. Hypotension, leukocytosis but no fever. For several days we look for a source but find nothing. Cultures only grow *Candida glabrata* in the urine and *Candida albicans* in the sputum. All other evaluations for a collection of pus to drain is negative. I want to find a source to control and can't find one.

Over the weekend the patient is started on intravenous caspofungin for the *Candida* in the urine, and when I return I scoff and sneer, since caspofungin has no urinary levels, so stop it. Still, after a dose of the caspofungin, the white blood cells took a dip towards normal.

The next day, I ponder. Two sites with *Candida*, total parenteral nutrition, broad-spectrum antibiotics, central line, diabetic, unexplained culture negative leukocytosis. Is this occult disseminated *Candida*? In olden times before the interwebs, when I used a TRS-80, about half of patients who died of *Candida* at autopsy had negative blood cultures antemortem. I am not sure that data applies in the modern era of high speed internets, MacBook Airs, and better culture media. Still, few organisms leave the blood for the tissues faster than a *Candida*, so I am never reassured by negative fungal blood cultures.

I had them call the ophthalpmolpogistps (I know there is a 'p' in that word somewhere, I am just not certain where it goes) as it is not uncommon for patients to have fungus balls in the back of the eyes when they have bloodstream *Candida* infections. Over the years I have made the diagnosis this way, but this time no dice. Besides calling the eye docs, and more a "what the hell" than any real conviction, I restart the caspofungin. But this time I send off a 1-3 beta-D-glucan, a test for invasive fungal infections that will take about 5 days to return.

Over the next few days the patients gets much better, a decrease in the white cell count, a resolution of the hypotension, and extubation. And today the beta glucan comes back way positive: 307. So disseminated *Candida* it is after all.

By the *Candida* score the patient was at risk, but at the time I restarted the caspofungin, it wasn't due to a great clinical insight. It was more, "Well, I don't know, maybe it's *Candida*, but let's treat while we wait on the blood test." At the time I could have decided to wait on the treatment; I usually lean that way. Right decision, but maybe more luck than skill. Still, there is no fate but what we make. I'll be back.

Rationalization

Crit Care Med. 2009 May;37(5):1624-33. Usefulness of the "Candida score" for discriminating between Candida colonization and invasive candidiasis in non-neutropenic critically ill patients: a prospective multicenter study. http://www.ncbi.nlm.nih.gov/pubmed/19325481

World J Surg. 2004 Jun;28(6):625-30. Combined assessment of beta-D-glucan and degree of candida colonization before starting empiric therapy for candidiasis in surgical patients. http://www.ncbi.nlm.nih.gov/pubmed/15366757

Lancet. 1995 Jan 7;345(8941):17-20. Plasma (1—>3)-beta-D-glucan measurement in diagnosis of invasive deep mycosis and fungal febrile episodes. http://www.ncbi.nlm.nih.gov/pubmed/7799700

Needle In a Needle Stack

ID is a low-tech subspecialty, at least most of the time. I do a history and physical, review the labs and x-rays and send off tests whose methodologies have been unchanged for years: cultures and serologies. We are so last century.

The promise of molecular testing has yet to be fulfilled. Although the occasional PCR or 16s ribosome assay has been of benefit, the cost, turnaround time, and sensitivity often render these tests onerous for acute care. Not much help if the test takes a couple of weeks to come back except to tell the pathologist at autopsy what the patient had.

The patient has renal failure due to polycystic kidney disease and is on continuous ambulatory peritoneal dialysis (CAPD). She presents with fevers, abdominal pain, and cloudy peritoneal fluid. CAPD peritonitis. Not so hard. Cultures are sent and antibiotics started and the patient gets mostly better. Mostly. Cultures, unfortunately, grow nothing, and her fluid clears. But pain and peripheral leukocytosis persist.

A CT scan of the abdomen shows what really are "too numerous to count" kidney cysts. Her kidney and liver really put the poly in polycystic. The question is, is one of these cysts infected? CT or ultrasound can't say, and I gave up on tagged white cell studies years ago.

So what to do? Better living through radiation. PET scans tend to be used to find malignancy, but they can find infections as well. PET scans find areas with lots of metabolism and infections are chock-a-block full of metabolism. Oncologists don't get to have all the fun.

"Among 389 identified patients with ADPKD, 33 (8.4%) had 41 episodes of cyst infection, including eight definite and 33 likely cas-

es. The incidence of cyst infections in patients with ADPKD was 0.01 episode per patient per year. Microbiological documentation was available for 31 episodes (75%), Escherichia coli accounting for 74% of all retrieved bacterial strains. Positron emission tomography scan proved superior to ultrasound, Computed tomography scan, and magnetic resonance imaging for the detection of infected cysts. Clinical efficacy of initial antibiotic treatment was noted in 71% of episodes. Antibiotic treatment modification was more frequently required for patients who were receiving initial monotherapy compared with those who were receiving bitherapy. Large (diameter >5 cm) infected cysts frequently required drainage."

So I ordered a PET scan and single, small, renal cyst glowed like Chernobyl. For years I have been trying to find a way to diagnose infected cysts and it looks like there is finally a reliable methodology.

The infected cyst was not amenable to drainage due to its location, so we pushed ahead with antibiotics and she slowly got better.

Rationalization

Transplant Proc. 2009 Jun;41(5):1942-5. Differentiation between infection in kidney and liver cysts in autosomal dominant polycystic kidney disease: use of PET-CT in diagnosis and to guide management.

http://www.ncbi.nlm.nih.gov/pubmed/19545761

Clin J Am Soc Nephrol. 2009 Jul;4(7):1183-9. Epub 2009 May 21. Cyst infections in patients with autosomal dominant polycystic kidney disease.

http://www.ncbi.nlm.nih.gov/pubmed/19470662

I Don't Cotton to That

I HAVE said in the past that IV drug use is not necessarily the most salubrious of lifestyles. Salubrious. A moist word, I drool when it speak it.

The patient is a user of heroin and injects a hit of H. 45 minutes later she has uncontrollable rigors and then a fever, and thence to the ER for admission.

History and physical reveals nothing else. Blood cultures are negative.

The usual pattern for fevers is an antigen interacts with macrophage, which makes tumor necrosis factor and some interleukins, which travels to the thalamus, which says "we are infected, red alert, we need a fever," so we get a reset of the temperature, a rigor (about 45 minutes have passed at this point), then a fever, then a sweat to break the fever. More than infection can set off this cascade.

Besides heroin being a rich microbiologic stew, and mixing with heroin with tap water, both good sources for antigens, sometimes the heroin is filtered through cotton to remove the larger debris before injection and that can lead to cotton fever.

"Cotton fever is a benign, self-limited syndrome that may mimic sepsis in intravenous drug addicts. We present an illustrative case and a review of the literature. Serious illness such as pneumonia and infectious endocarditis must always be considered in febrile addicts. However, trivial illness accounts for 16% to 26% of such fevers."

Sometimes cotton fever is not so benign. Cotton can he colonized with *Enterobacter agglomerans* and can lead to bacteremia and metastatic infections. Why does cotton have *Enterobacter agglomerans*? Stink bugs. Really. BTW: *Enterobacter* is now called

Pantoea.

"The southern green stink bug, Nezara viridula (L.), is a signif-icant pest of cotton, Gossypium hirsutum L., and is becoming an increasing challenge due to the decrease in use of broad-spectrum insecticides on the crop. The southern green stink bug can vector an opportunistic Pantoea agglomerans strain (designated Sc 1-R) into cotton bolls, resulting in infection."

Pantoea is found in the gastrointestinal tract of the stinkbug, so it is fever from injecting bug poo. *Pantoea* goes on to destroy cotton crops and cause the occasion human infection associated with penetrating trauma by vegetative material.

Lastly, Googling "cotton fever" to show the resident the liter-ature on the topic, I can across http://www.heroinhelper.com/, which offers all sorts of practical advice for having a quality her-oin experience, including how to avoid cotton fever.

I love ID. I am still amazed at the paths infections can take to get to me. Cotton fever, stinkbugs and heroin helper. Only in Infectious Disease.

Rationalization

J Emerg Med. 1990 Mar-Apr;8(2):135-9. Cotton fever": a benign fe-brile syndrome in intravenous drug abusers. http://www.ncbi.nlm.nih.gov/pubmed/2362114

Arch Intern Med. 1993 Oct 25;153(20):2381-2. Enterobacter ag-glomerans—associated cotton fever. http://www.ncbi.nlm.nih.gov/pubmed/8215743

J Econ Entomol. 2009 Feb;102(1):36-42. Temporal analysis of cotton boll symptoms resulting from southern green stink bug feeding and transmission of a bacterial pathogen. http://www.ncbi.nlm.nih.gov/pubmed/19253615

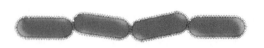

Concepts

How people conceptualize diseases and therapies determines their practices.

One of the classics of medicine is *Observations on spiraling empiricism: its causes, allure, and perils, with particular reference to antibiotic therapy*, an article everyone should read. It outlines the cognitive mistakes that physicians make in giving antibiotics, but it broadly applicable to all of medicine. Understanding cognitive errors and biases, and more importantly, watching for your own cognitive errors and biases, is key to being a good health care provider.

Still, I often think that many in health care consider infections more like demons that need exorcism than small life forms in need of extirpating. You can see examples in the language that people use to describe antibiotics. You know with 100% sensitivity and specificity that anyone who uses the terms "big gun," "strong" or "powerful" as adjectives to describe antibiotics is a moron who knows nothing about antibiotics. Sorry, did I say moron? I mean imbecile. But not an idiot.

There is nothing intrinsically strong, big gun, or powerful about antibiotics—those are advertising terms used to fool the prescriber into thinking that by giving a specific antibiotic they are giving the patient something special.

Here is a concept: how about giving the appropriate antibiotic; one that optimally kills the relevant bacteria in the infected space with the least toxicity, cost and resistance. Naw. That would require thought and understanding. Better to give, say, ertapenem "the Power of One" (I thought one was the loneliest number. Two can be as bad as one, it's the loneliest number since the number one) or Zosin, with a lightening bolt hitting the agar plate. Why worry about MICs and pharmacokinetics, when you can have the wrath of mighty Zeus smiting your bacteria?

This gets to the misbegotten cousin of antibiotic prescribing: the need to "double cover" *Pseudomonas.*

Combination antibiotics can be important: in sepsis (although the data are questionable) and empirically for some infections prior to getting the cultures back. If you give monotherapy and the patient's organism is resistant, mortality goes up. I rarely quibble about antibiotic choices in the first 48 hours of a patient's illness, since it is best to kill all the potential organisms up front. Combination therapy is useful pending cultures to CYA. However, once the data are back, narrow the antibiotics.

I saw a patient with probable hospital/ventilator-acquired pneumonia due to *Pseudomonas* who was much better on therapy: fever down, white blood cell count down, all systems heading towards improvement, and the primary team insisted that the patient be on "double coverage" for the *Pseudomonas.* I was the weekend cover guy, so I didn't throw a fit about it.

Data?

"Antibiotic combination using a fourth generation cephalosporin with either an aminoside or a fluoroquinolone is not associated with a clinical or biological benefit when compared to cephalosporin monotherapy against common susceptible pathogens causing VAP."

and

"Monotherapy in the treatment of Pseudomonas VAP has an excellent success rate in patients with trauma. Empiric monotherapy therapy should be modified once susceptibility of the microorganism is documented (all isolates were sensitive to cefepime) and antibiotic choice should be based on local patterns of susceptibilities. The routine use of combination therapy for synergy is unnecessary."

Combination therapy adds cost and toxicity and does not prevent the emergence of resistance (it may accelerate resistance, as one would predict if there is rudimentary understanding of microbiology and evolution). It does not, except in very specific cases, improve outcomes.

Not that people change practice based on the data. It only took 140 years for handwashing to become standard. Sigh. I seem to be a wee bit ranty today. Maybe I am reacting to yesterday being Blue Monday, the most depressing day of the year. And get off my lawn.

Rationalization

Am J Med. 1989 Aug;87(2):201-6. Observations on spiraling empiricism: its causes, allure, and perils, with particular reference to antibiotic therapy. http://www.ncbi.nlm.nih.gov/pubmed/2667357

A Medical-Skeptical Classic. http://www.sciencebasedmedicine.org/?p=388

Crit Care. 2006;10(2):R52. Combination therapy versus monotherapy: a randomised pilot study on the evolution of inflammatory parameters after ventilator associated pneumonia. http://www.ncbi.nlm.nih.gov/pubmed/16569261

J Trauma. 2009 Apr;66(4):1052-8; discussion 1058-9. Efficacy of monotherapy in the treatment of Pseudomonas ventilator-associated pneumonia in patients with trauma. http://www.ncbi.nlm.nih.gov/pubmed/19359914

....

Gimme That Old Time Diarrhea

I REMEMBER when there was no *C. difficile*, no *Helicobacter*, no HIV, no West Nile Virus. Simple times, with simple diseases, and cephalosporins had only two generations. Men were real men, women were real women, and antibiotic associated diarrhea was real antibiotic associated diarrhea.

So I get a call from an intern: the patient came in with real bad diarrhea after antibiotics, which is not as pleasant as the real good diarrhea. There are lots of white cells in the stool and the cultures grow MRSA. *C. difficile* is negative.

What, I am asked, do I make of that?

Sit down, my son, and listen to a story of the distant past, when pseudomembranous colitis was thought to be due to S. aureus. It is why we gave vancomycin for antibiotic associated colitis. Turns out we were doing the right thing for the wrong reason. But for a long time, we had no clue as to the etiologic bacteria, only that clindamycin was great at causing it.

"With the plethora of clinical, epidemiological, and laboratory information available from this symposium and numerous publications, the etiological mechanisms of colitis associated with clindamycin therapy should be readily apparent . The clues are tantalizing, but many of us remain perplexed. There is no apparent explanation for its unique pathology which is localized in the colon, its spotty epidemiological pattern as seen in various institutions , its relative benignity, and its curious similarities to the surgical-vascular disease of the past."

Now we know. Most cases were due to C. difficile. Most, but not all. Occasionally Staph will cause a severe inflammatory diarrhea. Usually it is after consumption of preformed S. aureus enterotoxins, not the organism, that leads to diarrhea. But sometimes people consume the organism and it can cause lots of diarrhea, in part mediated by the enterotoxins, although S. aureus makes more toxins than a Trailblazer team has arthroscopic surgeries. If you live in Portland, you understand and commiserate.

"Staphylococcus aureus has been implicated as a cause of antibiotic-associated diarrhea; however, reports rarely originate from the United States. We report 5 cases of antibiotic-associated diarrhea caused by methicillin-resistant S. aureus (MRSA). Eighty percent of the stool specimens were greenish. Heavy growth of MRSA from greenish stool culture may warrant oral vancomycin therapy."

I didn't ask the color of the poo. I just said treat. And the patient improved.

Rationalization

Eur J Gastroenterol Hepatol. 2005 Nov;17(11):1225-7. Postoperative methicillin-resistant Staphylococcus aureus enteritis following hysterectomy: a case report and review of the literature. http://www.ncbi.

nlm.nih.gov/pubmed/16215435

Int J Food Microbiol. 2000 Oct 1;61(1):1-10. Staphylococcal enterotoxins.
http://www.ncbi.nlm.nih.gov/pubmed/11028954

Diagn Microbiol Infect Dis. 2009 Apr;63(4):388-9. Epub 2009 Feb
18. Antibiotic-associated diarrhea due to methicillin-resistant Staphylococcus aureus.
http://www.ncbi.nlm.nih.gov/pubmed/19232861

J Infect Dis. 1977 Mar;135 Suppl:S89-94. Pseudomembranous enterocolitis: a review of its diverse forms. http://jid.oxfordjournals.org/
content/135/Supplement/S89.long Read the paper from 1977 where
they discuss all the potential etiologies, with no mention of Clostridia.

POLL RESULTS
I remember a time before

- cephalosporins 21%
- vaccinations 5%
- Medicare 14%
- EMR's 29%
- hand hygiene (last week at some hospitals) 24%
- Other Answers 7%
  1.   BLOGS
  2.   Salvarsan 606
  3.   CDs

Being Complete

WHEN I was a resident, one of the attendings wore a button that said "Be compulsive."

Eh. It is important, I know, but being compulsive does not come naturally to me. Be thorough. Be complete. That's more like it. Compulsive is a little too OCD a command for me.

I was asked to see a patient with a fever after a stroke. For three or four days before admission she had a declining and increasingly confused mental status on top of a baseline unreliability and combativeness. She refuses to take her medications for hypertension, diabetes and seizures, as they "do her no good." But still, for a stroke, it was a wee bit slow in onset.

The usual causes of fever were negative and the CT scan of the head showed a defect in the temporal-parietal area of the brain.

Fevers and a temporal-parietal lesion? Sounds like herpes simplex virus (HSV) to me. Although the CT did not look like a typical HSV lesion, the onset of symptoms were not like a stroke.

So I suggested, rather half-heartedly, to do a lumbar puncture, send it for HSV testing by polymerase chain reaction (PCR), and in the meantime start acyclovir.

And I will be damned if the HSV PCR on the spinal fluid was positive.

Could it be HSV reactivation from the trauma of a stroke? Not that I can find. If a stroke will cause a true positive but clinically unrelated reactivation of Herpes in the brain, it has yet to be reported on the PubMeds. There are some mouse models to suggest this could be possibility, but zero human data.

The fevers could be due to the stroke alone and HSV a red herring. Short of a brain biopsy, I will never know for sure.

I wish I had been more emphatic that HSV was the diagnosis, rather than going down the differential of fevers and tempo-ral-parietal brain necrosis. It would have made the result more impressive for my perspicacious diagnostic abilities.

But maybe I will get lucky with round 2. A second patient has plaques on her skin that I initially though were psoriasis, but did not have the shiny/flaky look typical of the disease. I knew she had been on a mental decline of late and is too young to be de-mented. Plus the MRI does not look like a dementing brain. The lumbar puncture? Protein 180, normal glucose, several hundred mixed cells. Could the plaques be lichenoid syphilis? And the dementia is syphilis as well?

Could be. This time I declared it to be syphilis and I will have the rapid plasma reagin results back tomorrow.

Update: It was negative. Of late it seems I make more diagno-sis from being complete rather than the flash of insight that is the more enjoyable way to come up with the diagnosis.

Oh well. As long as I get to the destination, does the journey matter? Yeah. It does.

Rationalization

J Virol. 1992 April; 66(4): 2150-2156 Rapid in vivo reactivation of herpes simplex virus in latently infected murine ganglionic neu-rons after transient hyperthermia. http://jvi.asm.org/cgi/content/ab-stract/66/4/2150

POLL RESULTS

I think

- It's the journey, not the destination. 23%
- It's the destination. 8%
- The ends justify the means. 3%
- Being right half the time beats being half-right all the time. 33%
- I'd rather be right than happy. 23%
- Other Answers 10%
    1.   I'd be happy if the destination was right and the journey was free.

2.   Its better to be lucky than good.

3.   It's the journey AND the destination that makes the probability of being > 1/2 right > 1/2 the time, and makes me happiest!

4.   I'd rather have a free bottle in front of me than a prefrontal lobotomy

A Bad Two Fer

A MIDDLE-AGED heroin user found unresponsive and clothed in a bathtub and transported to the hospital.

The white blood cell count is 36,000 cells per microliter. 4,000 to 11,000 is normal.

The exam is tremendous: multiple embolic events to the hands and feet, some red and small, some big and black. CT scan shows multiple emboli to the kidney and brain. A CT of the chest shows numerous round infiltrates, some of which are cavitating.

So by exam and x-rays the patient has both right-sided and left-sided endocarditis, and the transthoracic echocardiogram shows vegetations on the aortic valve and the tricuspid valve. So the echo confirms what we already knew.

Not my record. Although multivavular endocarditis is not common, i have seen one case where three valves were involved and there are reports of all four heart valves being involved.

One bug in the blood, bad. Two bugs? Worse.

The blood cultures grow MSSA and *E. coli*. Which bug on which valve? Both? I do not know. Again, not my record—which is three bugs in all the blood cultures, in the same patient that had three valves involved.

The world record, and I can't find the reference again (every time I look for this case report I can't find it), is, I think, a baker's dozen organisms in a German heroin user. Clot on valve is a hospitable environment for bacteria, and if you keep injecting bacteria with your heroin, the bacteria will pile on the clot like a bacillary scrum.

E. coli is a distinctly unusual as a cause of endocarditis, with a little over 100 cases in the literature on native valves.

"Review of the published literature yielded 127 cases with an overall mortality rate of 52%."

The patient cannot give a history, but I wonder if he uses toilet water to mix the drugs—a not uncommon occurrence since if you are withdrawing, the toilet stall gives both privacy and ready access to water to get a fix as rapidly as possible.

Toilet water, tap water, river water, Culligan water, puddle water, and spit, none of which are sterile, have all been used to mix heroin by at least one patient of mine over the years.

It is a credit to the host immune system and the lack of a landing site that we do not see more infections in intravenous drug users.

The moral equivalent in the hospital is injecting meds without a good cleaning of the IV hub. I wonder how many infections in the hospital we can blame on bacteria being pushed into the catheter with the medications.

"One hundred sixty-four cases (82 case pairs) were studied. We identified intraopera- tive bacterial transmission to the IV stopcock set in 11.5% (19/164) of cases, 47% (9/19) of which were of provider origin. We identified intraoperative bacterial transmission to the anesthesia environment in 89% (146/164) of cases, 12% (17/146) of which were of provider origin. The number of rooms that an attending anesthesiologist supervised simultaneously, the age of the patient, and patient discharge from the operating room to an intensive care unit were independent predictors of bacterial transmission events not directly linked to providers. CONCLUSION: The contaminated hands of anesthesia providers serve as a significant source of patient environmental and stopcock set contamination in the operating room."

Probably we will never know with certainty in clinical practice if the hub is the source of infection, but if you are injecting me and mine, you had damn well scrub the hub. I hope my healthcare worker has better technique than an IVDA. Or is that asking too much?

The patient did not survive, an unfortunate but common outcome of endocarditis in drug users.

Rationalization

Infectious Diseases in Clinical Practice: July 2010 - Volume 18 - Issue 4 - pp 247-250 Escherichia coli Endocarditis: A Case Report and Review of the Literature.

Hand contamination of anesthesia providers is an important risk factor for intraoperative bacterial transmission. Anesth Analg. 2011 Jan
http://www.ncbi.nlm.nih.gov/pubmed/20686007

POLL RESULTS
I
- always scrub the hub. 72%
- never scrub the hub, if I can't see it, it doesn't exist. 0%
- am sterile and have the urology/gyn report to prove it. 4%
- think gloves are enough, who needs to clean the hub. 12%
- if the the patient can't see that I am doing something wrong, then there isn't a problem. 12%
- Other Answers 0%

ID is Phat (as in hip hop venacular, not Marvel superheros. Well, maybe both.)

I HAVE a biased practice. Probably 95% of my patients are acutely ill and hospitalized, often trying to die. With the subset of patients I see, there may be a little confirmation bias, but I have a healthy respect for how infections can kill, or try to kill, people. Gotta respect the pathogen.

The patient is a middle-aged female with a renal transplant who has 24 hours of fevers and cough, and comes into the hospital and over the next 24 hours proceeds to intubation with a dense, bilateral hemorrhagic pneumonia.

The nasal wash is negative, but the bronchoscopy has influenza A, type pending, but I am betting on H1N1. It is a presentation like that described in the 1919 pandemic, with a rapid progression of hemorrhagic pneumonia which, in the pre-ICU era, usually meant a quick and horrible death. It is not a nice way to die.

A recent *Clinical Infectious Diseases* article postulated that the hemorrhagic pneumonia seen in 1918-1919 may have been due to aspirin use, which I do not know if the patient was taking—although if she was, I doubt it was at the doses recommended in 1919.

> *"...early deaths exhibited extremely "wet," sometimes hemorrhagic lungs. The hypothesis presented herein is that aspirin contributed to the incidence and severity of viral pathology, bacterial infection, and death, because physicians of the day were unaware that the regimens (8.0-31.2 g per day) produce levels associated with hyperventilation and pulmonary edema in 33% and 3% of recipients, respectively. Recently, pulmonary edema was found at autopsy in 46% of 26 salicylate-intoxicated adults. Experimentally, salicylates increase lung fluid and protein levels and impair mucociliary clearance. In 1918, the US Surgeon General, the US Navy, and the Journal of the American Medical Association recommended use of aspirin just before the October death spike. If these recommendations were followed, and if pulmonary edema occurred in 3% of persons, a significant proportion of the deaths may be attributable to aspirin."*

It may be the transplant medications that allowed the influenza run rampant, but I wonder more about the obesity, as she is about 3 times ideal body weight. The more overweight you are, the greater the chance of dying of influenza.

Obese people have elevated blood leptin levels, which is associated with increased mortality from infections in humans and animal models. Also, leptin levels are elevated in pregnancy, another group at increased risk for death from influenza.

So pregnancy and obesity may have a common physiologic pathway that leads to increased influenza mortality. But as is often the case in ID, the reason for the commonalty may lie deep in our evolutionary past. The

> *"...tuberculosis epidemic during previous centuries generated selective pressures that intensified the metabolic syndrome and the*

inflammatory processes now associated with obesity. These pro in-flammatory defenses (with immune systems that are especially ro-bust and more easily triggered) in partnership with the metabolic syndrome (insulin resistance, dyslipidemias, and hypertension), may have provided an advantage during the tuberculosis pan-demic when food availability was limited and average life span was short."

The physiology of obesity may have been protective against TB in pregnancy. But in a society with excess calories, it resulted in a tendency to pack on the adipose, leading to a primed pro-in-flammatory response and resultant increased mortality from in-fluenza. Evolving less morbidity from TB led to increased mor-tality from flu. Evolution giveth and evolution taketh away. At least I still have my appendix. Actually, I don't.

I keep saying this: ID is just so 42. I know I am horribly biased, but does any other area of medicine offer so many curiosities in so many other areas of life, the universe and everything? Nope.

Rationalization

Clin Infect Dis. 2009 Nov 1;49(9):1405-10. Salicylates and pandemic influenza mortality, 1918-1919 pharmacology, pathology, and historic evidence. http://www.ncbi.nlm.nih.gov/pubmed/19788357

Transpl Infect Dis. 2010 Apr;12(2):127-31. Epub 2010 Jan 20. Influ-enza A/H1N1 2009 pneumonia in kidney transplant recipients: char-acteristics and outcomes following high-dose oseltamivir exposure. http://www.ncbi.nlm.nih.gov/pubmed/20102550

Clin Infect Dis. 2011 Feb;52(3):301-12. Epub 2011 Jan 4. A novel risk factor for a novel virus: obesity and 2009 pandemic influenza A (H1N1). http://www.ncbi.nlm.nih.gov/pubmed/21208911

Evolutionary Speculation About Tuberculosis and the Metabolic and Inflammatory Processes of Obesity. JAMA. 2009;301(24):2586-2588. doi: 10.1001/jama.2009.930 http://jama.ama-assn.org/content/301/24/2586.extract

Lower Risk of Tuberculosis in Obesity. Arch Intern Med. 2007;167(12):1297-1304. http://archinte.ama-assn.org/cgi/content/abstract/167/12/1297

POLL RESULTS

The area of medicine more interesting than ID is
* what? 22%
* you must be kidding. 22%
* fugget aboutit. 11%
* no way. 11%
* you crazy if you add a suggestion to 'other'. 19%
* Other Answers 16%
  1.   Nitric oxide physiology
  2.   renal
  3.   iron justice and daedalus4U are both annoying
  4.   Pharmacy, obviously

An Evening Drink

So the patient and his roommate are sipping an evening apéritif when the patient has an unexpected loss of consciousness and a massive aspiration of stomach contents.

The patient is admitted to the ICU in acute respiratory distress and is intubated. A chest x-ray shows multilobar infiltrates and the patient has a therapeutic bronchoscopy on admission and the next day to remove the aspirated stomach contents from the lung. All the cultures grow yeast and it is identified as *Saccharomyces cerevisiae.*

Huh? Brewer's yeast in all the specimens. Real?

It is all in how you tell the history. The patients are prison cellmates, the apéritif is pruno and the unexpected loss of consciousness is due to an assault.

Pruno is, for those of you not in the know, per the ever-helpful Wikipedia

"... a prison wine, is an alcoholic liquid variously made from apples, oranges, fruit cocktail, ketchup, sugar, and possibly other ingredients, including bread. Pruno originated in (and remains largely confined to) prisons, where it can be produced cheaply, easily, and discreetly. The concoction can be made using only a plastic

bag, hot running water, and a towel or sock to conceal the pulp during fermentation. The end result has been colorfully described as a "vomit-flavored wine-cooler", although flavor is not the primary objective. Depending on the time spent fermenting, the sugar content, and the quality of the ingredients and preparation, pruno's alcohol content by volume can range from as low as 2% (equivalent to a very weak beer) to as high as 14% (equivalent to a strong wine)."

It gives you an idea how much people like alcohol when they will drink vomit-flavored wine-cooler, which to my way of thinking is all wine-coolers. Pruno has been a source of botulism when potato skins were used as one of the ingredients. In this case the pneumonia was probably caused by the massive inhalation of pruno containing *Saccharomyces cerevisiae*.

There is a case of pneumonia due to *Saccharomyces cerevisiae* reported in an AIDS patient. When I was a fellow I had an AIDS patient who was a home brewer who had the organism in his blood. I guess you say I know what "aled" him. I have also seen a pair of cases of *S. boulardii* fungemia due to probiotics given with/ for severe colitis.

Saccharomyces cerevisiae is an uncommon pathogen:

"We found 92 cases of Saccharomyces invasive infection. Predisposing factors were similar to those of invasive candidiasis, with intravascular catheter and antibiotic therapy being the most frequent. Blood was the most frequent site of isolation (for 72 patients). S. boulardii accounted for 51.3% of fungemias and was exclusively isolated from blood. Compared with patients infected with S. cerevisiae, patients infected with S. boulardii were more frequently immunocompetent and had a better prognosis. Saccharomyces invasive infection was clinically indistinguishable from an invasive candidiasis. Overall, S. cerevisiae clinical isolates exhibited low susceptibility to amphotericin B and azole derivatives. However, global outcome was favorable in 62% of the cases. "

The literature suggests voriconazole is the best antifungal, and the patient is slowly improving on this agent. Still, an odd way to get a *Saccharomyces cerevisiae* pneumonia. I will always prefer my *Saccharomyces cerevisiae* from a French Bordeaux or an Oregon IPA. There are many yeasts used to ferment wines, again from the Wikipedia:

> *"The most common genera of wild yeasts found in winemaking include Candida, Klöckera/Hanseniaspora, Metschnikowiaceae, Pichia and Zygosaccharomyces. Wild yeasts can produce high-quality, unique-flavored wines; however, they are often unpredictable and may introduce less desirable traits to the wine, and can even contribute to spoilage. Traditional wine makers, particularly in Europe, advocate use of ambient yeast as a characteristic of the region's terroir; nevertheless, many winemakers prefer to control fermentation with predictable cultured yeast. The cultured yeasts most commonly used in winemaking belong to the Saccharomyces cerevisiae (also known as "sugar yeast") species. "*

Candida? Really? No wonder why some wines taste like a diaper rash, not that I know what a diaper rash tastes like. Nonetheless, feel free to send me a case or two of a good French wine

---

Rationalization

J Clin Microbiol. 1989 Jul;27(7):1689-91. Saccharomyces cerevisiae pneumonia in a patient with acquired immune deficiency syndrome. http://www.ncbi.nlm.nih.gov/pubmed/2671026

Clin Infect Dis. 2005 Dec 1;41(11):1559-68. Epub 2005 Nov 1. Invasive Saccharomyces infection: a comprehensive review. http://www.ncbi.nlm.nih.gov/pubmed/16267727

POLL RESULTS
I prefer my yeast from

- beer 35%
- wine 29%
- bread 20%
- Vegemite 6%
- popcorn topping. So says the wikipedia on yeast. Blech. 6%

Curbsides

I WAS rounding at one of my many hospitals and overheard a conversation between a hospitalist and a specialist. The specialist was adamant that she could not and would not do a curbside, but would only offer general information about the condition, not specific answers to the question at hand. Specific information would require a consult.

It turns out that a member of her group had been found liable in a case where curbside advice was asked for and given and there was a bad outcome. The curbsiding physician had mentioned the curbsided physician's name in the chart and when the case went legal, the curbsided was found partly responsible. Evidently there has been more than one case of a doc being liable for the outcome of a curbside.

The devil is in the details, and I have none of the details, of the case, but it gives one (the one being me) pause. Curbsides are a large part of the day. I probably get a dozen curbsides and since I work in teaching hospitals, I can field numerous questions as I stroll the hospital halls.

I remember I once had a call from an intern at the start of the year. How long, she asked, do you treat a urinary tract infection? Three days. What's the bug? *Pseudomonas.*

Hmmm. I started asking questions. It turned out it was a septic diabetic renal transplant infection. Maybe three days would be a wee bit too short. The reply is only as good as the information given.

There was an abstract at the meetings several years ago (I can't find it) where a doc went and reviewed the chart and patient after a curbside and discovered he often gave bad advice to the curbsider due to inadequate information.

Curbsides are part of the free flow of knowledge that is important for patient care, and specialists often carry in their brain all sorts of obscure information that would be difficult, even in the era of the Googles, to find.

One study found

"A total of 1001 curbside consultations were fielded: 66% involved outpatients, and 97% were coded as initial consultations. A total of 78% of curbside consultations were considered complex in nature, being assigned a CPT code of level 4-5, including 84% of the inpatient and 75% of the outpatient curbside consultations. These curbside consultations would have generated 2480 wRVUs. During the same period, formal consultations generated 12,121 wRVUs. Thus, curbside consultations represented 17% (2480/14,601) of the clinical work value of the infectious diseases unit. If the infectious diseases unit had performed these curbside consultations as formal consultations, an additional $93,979 in revenue would have been generated."

$93,979? Whoa. One doc gives me a fine bottle of wine every year to say thank you for the time. I appreciate the thought. I'd rather have $93,979.

Others were not so impressed with the complexity of the cases in a curbside:

"A total three hundred and sixty-two such consultations were carried out during a three-month period. The ICs occurred most frequently in the hospital (82.3%). Most of the ICs from outside the hospital were by telephone. Most of the ICs (54.4%) were requested by fellows of specialists. 78.7% of the ICs were requested during working hours. 58.8% of consultations took less than 5 min, 18.8% took 6-10 min, 15.2% took 11-20 min, and 7.2% took over 20 min. The four most common reasons for obtaining ICs were to: help to select an appropriate treatment plan (41.4%), help to select an appropriate prophylaxis (19.3%), interpret laboratory data (10.2%), and provide information about antibiotics (10.2%). 30.1% of ICs resulted in subsequent formal consultation and only four patients (1.1%) were transferred to the consultants' clinics.

Informal consultations are a frequent occurrence in the practice of infectious diseases and clinical microbiology (ID&CM). Physicians use this sort of consultation to select an appropriate treatment plan and obtain medical information. This study confirms the importance of the ID&CM specialists as a resource for medical personnel."

My experience is a lot of curbsides represent trivial questions that would not seem to be time well spent as a formal consult (and my tux is in the cleaners). I really do not want to drive for half an hour to a hospital to OK linazolid for a MRSA abscess in a vancomycin- allergic patient.

It is a fine line. People need information and the curbside can be valuable. I can't be everywhere at once, despite a multiple personality disorder. Anyone want to talk to my goth cowgirl, or am I oversharing? And I do not want to be a diminutive of Richard if I am asked a question by a colleague. Much medical learning occurs informally talking with colleagues about specific cases. I am going to continue giving curbsides, but will be more circumspect about giving specific advice and bitch to the curbsiding doc that they damn well had better not quote me in the chart.

Rationalization

J Healthc Risk Manag. 2008;28(1):27-9. Minimizing the legal risk with 'curbside' consultation. http://www.ncbi.nlm.nih.gov/pubmed/20200900

Clin Infect Dis. 2010 Sep 15;51(6):651-5. The complexity, relative value, and financial worth of curbside consultations in an academic infectious diseases unit. http://www.ncbi.nlm.nih.gov/pubmed/20687842

Clin Microbiol Infect. 2003 Jul;9(7):724-6. Informal consultations in infectious diseases and clinical microbiology practice. http://www.ncbi.nlm.nih.gov/pubmed/12925117

Curbside Consult. http://www.sma.org.sg/sma_news/3801/infectious_ak.pdf

POLL RESULTS
Curbsides

- I get them freely and don't worry about the liability. 0%
- I give them freely and don't worry about the liability. 6%
- A bottle of wine? Maybe my ID consultant should get a case of French Bordeaux. 11%
- No one has ever asked me a question at the curb of a street. But hallside sounds wrong. 22%
- are GIGO. Garbage in, garbage out. If you want my opinion, get a consult. 50%
- Other Answers 11%
  1.   No one listens to me anyway

  2.   I am a hospitalist and when i get a curbside, i NEVER write the consultant's name in chart... unless they are mean to me.

Smattering

WORK is actually lacking in fascinomas. The cases have been quickies, no great diagnostic or therapeutic decisions. But there are curiosities nonetheless.

Today's patient underwent a catheterization (cath) for coronary artery disease, which is the usual reason I suppose. Stents were placed. I don't keep up on the indications for a cardiac cath. When I took care of these patients a quarter of a century ago, it was done for chest pain. Any chest pain. If the patient came in to the ER after moving a CHEST to get to their PAINE Webber files, they got a cath. Or so it seemed at the time. I probably exaggerate; I suppose my readers will set me straight.

Three days later the patient has fevers and rigors and comes back to the hospital, and has MRSA in the blood.

Nothing on exam, the cath site appears uninfected and there is nothing to suggest an infected groin pseudoaneurysm, a complication of cardiac cath that I have seen in the past. In order to perform the cath, a thin, flexible tube is inserted into the femoral artery in the groin and threaded through the blood vessels to the heart. A pseudoaneurysm can happen if blood leaks and pools outside the punctured femoral artery.

Could it be the stents? There are a smattering of infections reported involving cardiac stents and

> *"when infected, they are associated with the formation of intra-coronary abscesses and pseudoaneurysms with possible vessel thrombosis and ischaemic compromise of the heart."*

Not good.

He gets an echocardiogram and there is a big vegetation of the aortic valve.

Huh. Endocarditis. Expected given that *S. aureus* is the blood for no good reason is always endocarditis, but why?

Given the trauma of the cath bouncing against the valve and frequency of bacteremia, is a cath a risk for endocarditis?

Yeah, another smattering of cases.

Some vancomycin and the patient is getting better.

A curiosity and two smatterings. Best I can do today.

Rationalization

Infected pseudoaneurysm involving a drug-eluting stent. Interact Cardiovasc Thorac Surg. 2011 Jan 12. http://www.ncbi.nlm.nih.gov/pubmed/21228044

Staphylococcus lugdunensis endocarditis after angiography. Polenakovik H, Herchline T, Bacheller C, Bernstein J. Mayo Clin Proc. 2000 Jun;75(6):656-7. No abstract available.

Chest. 1976 Aug;70(2):293-6. Bacterial endocarditis after cardiac catheterization. http://www.ncbi.nlm.nih.gov/pubmed/947697

Facial Cellulitis?

TODAY I saw a 49-year-old male who has recurrent facial cellulitis.

He has had six outbreaks in the last 4 years, each on the right cheek. It originally started after a splash while cleaning a public restroom, which was aggressively cleaned. The splash, that is. It starts with tingling, then it becomes red, hot and swollen.

Multiple courses of both intravenous and oral antibiotics have been tried and the infection is always slow to respond, taking weeks to get better. He has also had variety of decontamination procedures without effect.

Physical exam shows a red patch, not tender, under the right eye/cheek. No skin breakdown. It looks more like an acute punch than an acute cellulitis.

No other past medical history. No fever and with normal labs.

What to do? I was intrigued by the tingling that preceded each cellulitis and sent a culture for herpes simplex virus (HSV), which grew HSV-2. I have seen HSV just about everywhere on the skin acting like cellulitis, including one patient who had it just between the shoulder blades. Not everything that looks like cellulitis is cellulitis, and the atypical features may tip you off as to an alternative diagnosis.

My hypothesis is that he got it from kiss from his girlfriend, who has cold sores, and not the work exposure. The timing is right and neither had any clinical HSV before. It is good to remember that while 1 in 5 Americans are seropositive for HSV-2, less than 10% have ever had active ulcers, yet are frequently excreting small amounts of virus. One never knows the true infectious provenance of a potential partner.

The question does come up: can you get an STD from a toilet

seat, and I usually reply only if you have sex in a stall. Ick. The data concerning toilets and STDs is surprisingly sparse, given the frequency with which this is used as an explanation on the web and elsewhere. Hot tubs are the closest you can get to a model

"Cutaneous bacterial infections, most commonly caused by Pseudomonas aeruginosa, have been clearly linked to use of hot tubs. A 10-year-old female with atopic eczema developed eczema herpeticum after hot tub use with a friend who had "fever blisters"; herpes simplex virus was recovered from cutaneous vesicles. Since herpesvirus has been shown to survive in the hot tub environment, herpes simplex should be considered as another potential cause of disease in the spa setting."

Most of the time it probably requires more active participation to acquire an infection.

"Pseudomonas aeruginosa acute prostatitis and urosepsis after sexual relations in a hot tub. We report a case of a previously healthy 38-year-old male with acute prostatitis and concurrent Pseudomonas aeruginosa urosepsis. Pulsed-field gel electrophoresis analysis confirmed that the source of the organism was the patient's newly purchased hot tub, which was filled with water from a stream."

Still, before getting into a public hot tub, maybe think about that famous love scene from *The Naked Gun*.

Rationalization

J Clin Microbiol. 2009 May;47(5):1607-8. Epub 2009 Mar 18. Pseudomonas aeruginosa acute prostatitis and urosepsis after sexual relations in a hot tub.

Pediatr Dermatol. 1985 Jul;2(4):322-3. Is eczema herpeticum associated with the use of hot tubs?

Ann Intern Med. 2005 Jan 4;142(1):47-55. Narrative review: diseases that masquerade as infectious cellulitis.

Bias

EVERYONE has their biases. I have mine. One is that I am a beta-lactam fan boy. If I can, I give a beta-lactam, and if I can, it's a penicillin or a cephalosporin, especially the first generations. I grew up before them-there high flautin' quinolones and beta lactamase inhibitors. I was a resident when moxilactam, the first third-generation cephalosporin, was released.

The patient is a diabetic who is admitted with cellulitis of the leg. Nothing at all unusual about the diagnosis. He is treated with vancomycin and, after a skin swab grows MSSA, he is sent home on clindamycin. At a follow-up visit in the clinic, the leg was worse, so he was admitted again for further IV antibiotics and they call me 2 days later.

I see a leg with a lot of subcutaneous blood, but most of the redness resolves with elevation. I think the infection is gone and most of the redness is post-infectious edema. Was that the case in the clinic? I do not know. It is not mentioned whether or not the leg was evaluated in the dependent position. If I have said it once, I have said it one time, you cannot evaluate the response to antibiotic of a cellulitic leg if it is in the dependent position. You have to position the leg higher than the heart and see if the redness remains with elevation. Of course, that technique doesn't work with Nick Chopper. I have cured innumerable (counting is not my strong point) cases of persisting cellulitis with elevation.

So I lift the leg higher than the heart. Poof. All the redness is gone. It's magic.

The other issue is the clindamycin. My bias is that clindamycin should not be used for *S. aureus* if you have another option like, um, I dunno, a beta-lactam? I know of no data to support that assertion, but my bias—and again it is a bias—is that if an antibiotic would not be used for my mother's MSSA prosthetic valve endocarditis, then don't use it. Sure, you will get away with it most of the time. But why practice medicine you can get away with?

Another bias of mine, not widely shared, is never use a third-generation cephalosporin for a *S. aureus* infection for convenience over a first generation. It is not as good. My bias was recently confirmed.

"Empirical treatment with cloxacillin or cefazolin (n=131) was associated with lower 30-day mortality as compared with cefuroxime (n=98, P=0.058), ceftriaxone or cefotaxime (n=194, p=0.008) and beta-lactam-beta-lactamase combinations (n = 61, p=0.013), with adjusted odds ratios (OR) for death ranging from 1.98 to 2.68. Definitive treatment with cefazolin (n=72) was not significantly different from cloxacillin (n=281); adjusted OR for 90-day mortality 0.91 (95% confidence interval 0.47-1.77). Treatment with cefazolin both in the empirical and definitive periods was not significantly different from cloxacillin; adjusted OR 0.81 (95% confidence interval 0.18-3.62). Treatment of MSSA bacteriemia with cefazolin is not significantly different from treatment with cloxacillin, while treatment with other beta-lactams, including second and third generation cephalosporins, might be associated with higher mortality."

Ha. I have been right all along. Again, my approach is that if a drug is not optimal for worst-case scenario, why use it elsewhere if you don't have to?

This patient probably needs mostly elevation and some oral cephalexin, and should get better.

And so it was.

Rationalization

Clin Microbiol Infect. 2010 Nov 13. doi: 10.1111/j.1469-0691.2010.03425.x. Are all beta-lactams similarly effective in the treatment of methicillin-sensitive Staphylococcus aureus bacteriemia? http://www.ncbi.nlm.nih.gov/pubmed/21073629

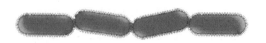

More Than the Usual Shingles?

THE patient is an elderly (late 80's) male with little in the way of past medical history.

He gets shingles across three dermatomes: T1, T2 and T3. Better than a T-101 or T-800, if you remember your *Terminator*, but unpleasant nonetheless. He did remember having chickenpox 70 years ago. I remember my case of chickenpox and we have super 8 film of me running around with the pox. So cute.

There is nothing odd about a case of zoster, except, perhaps, the epidemiology.

It used to be that we wallowed in childhood diseases. We would get infected, then our kids would get infected, and then our grandkids would get infected, and we would be exposed to varicella zoster virus and our antibody would get boosted. That is not happening, since kids are getting the vaccine and so older generations are not being exposed and their immunity is waning. One would think of that were the case, then there may be an increase in cases of shingles. Obviously a big pharma plot to increase the utilization of their vaccine, making it easier to insert those tracking nanobots.

And that is what is happening. In the old days,

"The probability of having had an attack of shingles before age 45 years is 8.6% for males and 10.5% for females, The risk of acquiring shingles over an expected lifetime (assuming no preventive vaccination) for males aged 45 years is 22% and for females 32%."

Now a recent CID article did show that zoster rates are going up, but they did not find evidence that it was due to the vaccine program.

"HZ incidence increased for the entire study period and for all

age groups, with greater rates of increase 1993-1996 (P < .001). HZ rates were higher for females than males throughout the study period (P < .001) and for all age groups (P < .001)...

Age-specific HZ incidence did not differ between adults residing in states with high varicella vaccine coverage and those in low-coverage states (P = .3173 for difference in incidence), but it was lower in children living in high-coverage states (P < .001). HZ incidence was lower in adults aged 20–50 years with dependents aged ≤12 years compared with adults without dependents (P < .01), but became similar over time."

I am not certain I buy it that the vaccine program does not affect the zoster rates. Although their data did not support the fact, there are methodological issues as the authors note, and there is as of yet no competing explanation for why the rates are increasing. At issue would be both rates of chickenpox in communities and exposures to adults to kids with chickenpox, not part of the study design.

"There were particular limitations in our analysis of the impact of varicella exposure on HZ incidence."

and

"Just why, then, are HZ rates increasing? This question is closely related to the broader question of why one-third of the population experiences HZ during their lifetimes [1], but two-thirds do not. Only a small portion of persons who experience HZ are immunosuppressed, suggesting that unrecognized risk factors are at play. We cannot know why HZ incidence is increasing if we cannot know how key risk factors for HZ are changing. Less well-defined factors that may play roles include comorbid chronic conditions, trauma, psychological stress, race, and family history [3, 8, 38–40]; however, the attributable risk associated with these factors is unlikely to be large or to have changed dramatically over time."

The only thing that has changed is the herd exposure to wild chickenpox. So, from basic principals, I would be inclined to attribute the increase to a lack of exposure to the antigens, indirectly supported by the benefit in the prevention of zoster by the elder who get the "shingles vaccine."

"The number of herpes zoster cases among vaccinated individuals was 828 in 130,415 person-years (6.4 per 1000 person-years; 95% confidence interval [CI], 5.9-6.8), and for unvaccinated individuals it was 4606 in 355,659 person-years (13.0 per 1000 person-years; 95% CI, 12.6-13.3). In adjusted analysis, vaccination was associated with a reduced risk of herpes zoster (hazard ratio [HR], 0.45; 95% CI, 0.42-0.48); this reduction occurred in all age strata and among individuals with chronic diseases. Risk of herpes zoster differed by vaccination status to a greater magnitude than the risk of unrelated acute medical conditions, suggesting results for herpes zoster were not due to bias. Ophthalmic herpes zoster (HR, 0.37; 95% CI, 0.23-0.61) and hospitalizations coded as herpes zoster (HR, 0.35; 95% CI, 0.24-0.51) were less likely among vaccine recipients."

Still, there is a lot yet to be learned about the epidemiology of shingles in the post-vaccination era. Maybe something else is going on, but I am skeptical that they proved the case it was not vaccination that is partly the etiology.

The patient developed some disseminated lesions as well, but clinically was fine. He has no immunodeficiency we can identify and will have to credit the disease to age.

Rationalization

The incidence of shingles and its implications for vaccination policy. Vaccine. 2003 Jun 2;21(19-20):2541-7. http://www.ncbi.nlm.nih.gov/pubmed/12744889
Clin Infect Dis. 2011 Feb;52(3):332-40. Herpes zoster incidence among insured persons in the United States, 1993-2006: evaluation of impact of varicella vaccination. http://www.ncbi.nlm.nih.gov/pubmed/21217180
JAMA. 2011 Jan 12;305(2):160-6. Herpes zoster vaccine in older adults and the risk of subsequent herpes zoster disease. http://www.ncbi.nlm.nih.gov/pubmed/21224457

Creep. Hip Hop or Alt?

So I creep yeah
Just keep it on the down low
Said nobody is supposed to know
So I creep yeah
'Cause he doesn't know
What I do and no attention
Goes to show oh so I creep. —TLC

THE patient has Streptococcus pneumoniae meningitis and bacteremia. Nothing too peculiar about the presentation and treatment.

The patient does have Systemic Lupus Erythematosis (SLE), and patients with SLE do not handle S. pneumoniae as well as normal people. Due to low complement levels, they are unable to opsonize (surround the bacteria with complement) as well as those with intact immune systems.

"RESULTS: The proportion of bacteria positive for C3b/iC3b was significantly lower in serum from patients with SLE (strain D39: 60.3% +/- s.e.m. 2.87, strain Io11697: 55.3% +/- 3.8) compared with healthy controls (strain D39: 70.6% +/- 2.0, P = 0.01; strain Io11697: 67.8% +/- 2.6; P = 0.05) and non-SLE rheumatic controls (strain D39: 69.8% +/- 3.1; P = 0.03). For the patients with SLE, there was no association between C3b/iC3b deposition and serum complement levels or measurable classical pathway activity. C3b/iC3b deposition on S. pneumoniae was significantly lower in serum from SLE patients with a past history of pneumonia (n = 3) compared with those without (n = 27; P = 0.03). CONCLUSIONS: Opsonization of S. pneumoniae with C3b/ iC3b was significantly reduced in serum from patients with SLE compared with non-SLE rheumatic disease and healthy controls. Failure to appropriately activate the immune system via comple-

ment may contribute to the increased susceptibility of SLE subjects to infections, and may correlate with a risk of pneumonia in a subgroup of SLE patients."

For some reason, maybe because it was a Medical Knowledge Self-Assessment Program (MKSAP) question from twenty years ago, I had assumed that SLE and meningitis went together like a condom and Left Eye. There is a hodgepodge of odd invasive pneumococcal infections in patients with SLE, such as cellulitis. Lupus is mentioned as a risk for pneumococcal meningitis, but whether it is due to the therapies or the disease itself I cannot tell.

This particular strep showed a mean inhibitory concentration (MIC) to penicillin of 0.19, so it was resistant to penicillin for the treatment of meningitis. The MIC to ceftriaxone was 0.25, so that antibiotic was still available. It is all in the relative concentrations: you want antibiotic levels in the CSF at least 10x the MIC when you treat meningitis. Penicillin doesn't get all that much into the CSF, even with inflammation. At least I do not have to give chloramphenicol, like I did in the old days.

Pneumococcal MIC to penicillin had been creeping up (see, I worked the initial lyrics into the essay) until the pneumococcal vaccine became available. The vaccine targeted the most common strains, which were also the more resistant strains, which has lead to a decrease in resistant pneumococcal disease. For a while the creeping resistance was halted, but no ecologic niche goes unfilled, and of late pneumococcal strains not covered by the vaccine were increasing in both frequency and resistance.

"Yearly resistance prevalence to most antibiotics had been increasing in the period 1996-2001. Adjusted prevalence rates in a multivariate model declined in the period 2001-2004 for penicillin, erythromycin, amoxicillin/clavulanate, trimethoprim/sulfamethoxazole, tetracycline, ceftriaxone, and multidrug. These same antibiotics showed a significant rebound for the period 2004-2007, with the largest overall increase for erythromycin, followed by amoxicillin/clavulanate, tetracycline, multidrug, penicillin, trimethoprim/sulfamethoxazole, and ceftriaxone. Changes in both decline and rebound were more marked for children <5 years old and for otitis media isolates."

and

"BACKGROUND: The pneumococcal conjugate vaccine (PCV7), introduced in February 2000, covered 82% of the U.S. pediatric population in 2005. Changes over time in serogroup prevalence and multidrug-resistance (MR) to antimicrobials were evaluated using the U.S. SENTRY surveillance program. METHODS: The study included 704 U.S. isolates, with equal numbers before (1998-1999) and after the introduction of the vaccine (2003-2004). Demographic data, serotype, and resistance profiles for five antimicrobial classes were analyzed. Strains displaying resistance to >or=2 classes were considered MR. Statistical analysis was performed using logistic regression. RESULTS: Prevalence of PCV7 serotypes was 68.5% in the prevaccine years, dropping to 29.3% in the postvaccine period. Among PCV7 serotypes, only 19F persisted, with nonvaccine (NV) serotype 19nonF strains increasing from 3% to 20% of total p<0.001. NV serotypes were 1.9 times (95% confidence interval [CI] 1.1-3.1) more likely to acquire MR over time. Although PCV7 serotypes constituted 84% of all MR isolates in the prevaccine era, MR was unchanged in the postvaccine period due to increased prevalence and acquisition of resistance by NV serotypes. MR among invasive isolates did not change over time, but increased among noninvasive NV isolates by 17% (95% CI 12-22%)."

Crap. I knew it was too good to last. Curse you, Mr. Darwin. The patient also works with young children, and she noted it has been a snotfest this year in the classroom. The kids are probably the vectors for infections in the adults.

But I'm a creep
I'm a pneumococcus
What the hell am I doing here?
I don't belong here
I don't care if it hurts
I want to have control
I want a perfect infection
I want a perfect soul.

Radiohead. Sort of.

Rationalization

Rheumatology (Oxford). 2009 Dec;48(12):1498-501. Epub 2009 Sep 30. Impaired C3b/iC3b deposition on Streptococcus pneumoniae in serum from patients with systemic lupus erythematosus. http://www.ncbi.nlm.nih.gov/pubmed/19797312

Microb Drug Resist. 2009 Dec;15(4):261-8. The impact of the pneumococcal conjugate vaccine on antimicrobial resistance in the United States since 1996: evidence for a significant rebound by 2007 in many classes of antibiotics. http://www.ncbi.nlm.nih.gov/pubmed/19857132

Microb Drug Resist. 2008 Jun;14(2):101-7. Serotype replacement and multiple resistance in Streptococcus pneumoniae after the introduction of the conjugate pneumococcal vaccine. http://www.ncbi.nlm.nih.gov/pubmed/18491947

When I ask my kids about who did "Creep" my youngest said: "Being edgy again, Dad?" Sigh.

All That Glows Is Not Cancer

BESIDES taking care of patients with acute infectious diseases, I have chaired the Infection Control programs at my hospitals for over 20 years. So I get the occasional calls about what to do when potential communicable diseases get admitted.

I get a call about a patient who had a growing lung nodule on CT, found incidentally. Secondhand smoke was her only cancer risk factor. Over time the nodule grew and it was positioned such that it was not easily amenable to either a percutaneous biopsy or a bronchoscopic biopsy. So a PET scan was obtained and the nodule glowed like Chernobyl. Tumor, right? You know the answer. Since you are reading an ID book, the category is probably not going to be "Cancer for 200, Alex." And you would be right.

The patient goes off to the OR for a resection and rather than tumor it is full of acid-fast bacilli and granuloma.

The patient has no risk factors for TB, except being human, which is often the only risk factor that is needed.

So I am asked, is she infectious post=op?

Probably not, I conclude. The infection is now in pathology. And sputum stains for acid-fast bacilli are reassuringly negative.

Is it going to be TB? Eh. Probably not. For now we wait before getting all twitter-pated (nothing to do with 140 characters) about a potential nosocomial TB exposure.

And it turned out to be *Mycobacterium avium-intracellulare*, aka MAI.

So did she need the surgery? Good question. I have had a horrible track record in treating MAI pneumonia. Lots of expensive antibiotics and side effects with never a cure. I tend to think that it is a surgical infection if you really want to cure it, but having part of a lung out is not a trivial intervention.

The literature supports lousy response and frequent side effects when treating MAI in the lung. Success rates average about 50%-ish, depending on the drugs used and the form of MAI pneumonia the patient has; there are at least 4 clinical patterns of the disease. Better than my outcomes to date.

This is not the first time a PET scan has been used to diagnose an MAI nodule. The nodule is often thought to be a malignancy, with the true diagnosis being made serendipitously in the OR. In parts of the world where TB is more common, PET scans are evidently being used diagnostically and to help determine extent of disease.

"Few studies have compared the clinical and radiographic findings of tuberculomas to those of solitary pulmonary nodules (SPNs) caused by Mycobacterium avium complex (MAC). We retrospectively analyzed clinical and radiographic findings from 26 patients with tuberculomas and 15 patients with SPNs caused by MAC. Median SPN size was 22 mm. In 26 patients (63%), the SPN was detected during a routine health checkup or evaluation of organs other than lungs. Patients with SPNs due to MAC were slightly older (median = 59 years) compared with those with tuberculomas (median = 50 years; P = 0.044). When we compared computed tomography (CT) features between patients with tuberculomas and patients with MAC, no significant differences

were found in SPN location or the presence of calcification, cavitation, central low attenuation, and the satellite lesions. Although the maximum standardized uptake values were slightly higher in patients with SPNs due to MAC (median = 8.5) compared with those with tuberculomas (median = 2.2), this difference was not significant (P = 0.053). Of the 15 patients with SPNs due to MAC, 10 were initially diagnosed with "tuberculoma" and administered antituberculosis medication. MAC pulmonary disease should be considered in the differential diagnosis of SPNs, even when encountered in geographic regions with a high prevalence of pulmonary tuberculosis."

One group used the PET to follow response to therapy. Kind of pricey; I would just ask the patient how their cough was doing. I wonder if MAI is sensitive to radiation. Maybe they just nuked it.

Rationalization

Chest. 2006 Oct;130(4):1234-41. The expanding spectrum of Mycobacterium avium complex-associated pulmonary disease. http://www.ncbi.nlm.nih.gov/pubmed/17035461

Mycobacterium avium complex Pulmonary Disease in Patients Without HIV Infection. CHEST August 2004 vol. 126 no. 2 566-581 http://chestjournal.chestpubs.org/content/126/2/566.full

Clin Nucl Med. 2009 Nov;34(11):818-20. PET scanning used for monitoring treatment response in Mycobacterium avium complex infection mimicking malignancy. http://www.ncbi.nlm.nih.gov/pubmed/19851186

Lung. 2010 Jan-Feb;188(1):25-31. Epub 2009 Dec 3 Solitary pulmonary nodules caused by Mycobacterium tuberculosis and Mycobacterium avium complex.

Don't Ask, But You Will Receive Anyway

I AM not prone to superstition and woo. I do not believe in ghosts or psychic abilities or homeopathy. I am from the reality-based community, knock on wood. But I wonder sometimes. Perhaps the Secret is true, kinda of sorta.

Of course, here is where I disappear into the morass of confirmation bias. It appears that when I read an article on a topic that is either new, or unusual in my practice, I see a case shortly thereafter. Woo woo, spooky.

I rarely see chronic diarrhea in the clinic, but this week I saw a middle-aged male who has had diarrhea and cramps for 15 years. It started with a trip to South America, where he developed a bad case of gastroenteritis. Since that time his bowels have not been normal. Loose stools and cramps now predominate, especially in the morning.

Interestingly, the symptoms resolve with a course of ciprofloxicin and relief persists for about a month or two after cessation of the antibiotics. Work-up over the years has been negative for numerous bacterial cultures and parasites, and he has had a normal colonoscopy.

There are numerous articles on the PubMeds on irritable bowel syndrome (IBS) following traveler's diarrhea.

"...we found that an episode of traveler's diarrhea was associated with a quintuple risk of developing irritable bowel syndrome."

Just last week I read an article in the *New England Journal of Medicine* on how rifaximin, an antibiotic used for traveler's diarrhea, can ameliorate the symptoms of IBS.

"Significantly more patients in the rifaximin group than in the placebo group had adequate relief of global IBS symptoms during

the first 4 weeks after treatment (40.8% vs. 31.2%, P=0.01, in TARGET 1; 40.6% vs. 32.2%, P=0.03, in TARGET 2; 40.7% vs. 31.7%, P<0.001, in the two studies combined). Similarly, more patients in the rifaximin group than in the placebo group had adequate relief of bloating (39.5% vs. 28.7%, P=0.005, in TARGET 1; 41.0% vs. 31.9%, P=0.02, in TARGET 2; 40.2% vs. 30.3%, P<0.001, in the two studies combined). In addition, significantly more patients in the rifaximin group had a response to treatment as assessed by daily ratings of IBS symptoms, bloating, abdominal pain, and stool consistency. The incidence of adverse events was similar in the two groups."

There are no randomized clinical trials of ciprofloxicin for the treatment of IBS, but anecdotes (the plural of anecdote is anecdotes, not data) suggest some efficacy.

So I think it is a post-infectious IBS mitigated with ciprofloxicin, mostly since I can't come up with an alternative explanation

I never see chronic diarrhea; it usually goes (and goes) to the GI docs. But I read an article on the topic, and the Universe presents me a case shortly thereafter. I really need to read an article about an ID doc winning the lottery.

Rationalization

Clin Infect Dis. 2005 Dec 1;41 Suppl 8:S577-86. Sequelae of traveler's diarrhea: focus on postinfectious irritable bowel syndrome. http://www.ncbi.nlm.nih.gov/pubmed/16267722

Clin Infect Dis. 2006 Oct 1;43(7):898-901. Epub 2006 Aug 25. Is traveler's diarrhea a significant risk factor for the development of irritable bowel syndrome? A prospective study. http://www.ncbi.nlm.nih.gov/pubmed/16941373

N Engl J Med. 2011 Jan 6;364(1):22-32. Rifaximin therapy for patients with irritable bowel syndrome without constipation. http://www.ncbi.nlm.nih.gov/pubmed/21208106

Dig Dis Sci. 2008 Jan;53(1):169-74. Epub 2007 May 23. Rifaximin versus other antibiotics in the primary treatment and retreatment of bacterial overgrowth in IBS. http://www.ncbi.nlm.nih.gov/pubmed/17520365

POLL RESULTS

When I read an journal article

- I see a case shortly thereafter. 3%
- I never see a case of anything odd I read about. 3%
- I don't read journals, I get all my information from this blog. 52%
- I only see cases of topics I do not read about. 6%
- I just wish for Tinkerbell to get better (who the wikipedia notes is a 'fictional character'). 21%
- Other Answers 15%

  1. I usually catch whatever I read about a week later.

  2. when I hear about science on the radio I often get a question about it soon after. NPR Rocks!

  3. I try to think how it relates to nitric oxide.

  4. I immediately get the symptoms.

··

See It While You Still Can

I AM an adult ID doc, more who I take care of rather than how I act. As such there are diseases I do not see. Otitis media, strep throat and acne are not issues that are a source of inpatient hospital consultation. Which is good. Can you imagine if acne needed my consultation? Whoa.

Respiratory syncytial virus (RSV) is mostly a disease of children, or so I thought. A bone marrow patient is admitted with mild shortness of breath and cough of 5 days duration. He has a bronchoscopy and they test the pulmonary secretions for everything. Really. I think there was no class of organism not looked for.

This year they have started doing a PCR panel that in one fell swoop tests for influenza A, B, and RSV. And his RSV was positive. So they called me.
RSV is often a bad disease in transplant patients, with a high mortality rate.

> "*The chest radiographs generally revealed diffuse patchy infiltrates, including alveolar opacities. Histology demonstrated diffuse alveolar damage, bronchiolitis with organizing pneumonia, and hyaline membrane formation. Over half required intubation, and 55% died. Although ribavirin therapy may be beneficial in some intubated patients, its overall efficacy cannot be established from this series.*"

In this case it was a mild disease with minimal infiltrates and fever. I think he may have acquired RSV from one of his grandchildren. The patient did fine with supportive care and intravenous immunoglobulin (IVIG). I suspect that it was not his first exposure to RSV given how mild his disease was. Inhaled ribavirin was not needed and it turns out the drug costs 4000 dollars a vial, or at that price, a vile, and we have no supplies available.

A quick search revealed that we had three adult patients in-house with RSV. I do not know how many are out-house. The Centers for Disease Control website suggests RSV is booming in the state, with 40 cases a week, mostly in kids. The same is true across the US. RSV occasionally causes disease in adults, but I do not look very often, since there is no therapy.

*"A total of 608 healthy elderly patients and 540 high-risk adults were enrolled in prospective surveillance, and 1388 hospitalized patients were enrolled. A total of 2514 illnesses were evaluated. RSV infection was identified in 102 patients in the prospective cohorts and 142 hospitalized patients, and influenza A was diagnosed in 44 patients in the prospective cohorts and 154 hospitalized patients. **RSV infection developed annually in 3 to 7 percent of healthy elderly patients** and in 4 to 10 percent of high-risk adults. Among healthy elderly patients, RSV infection generated fewer office visits than influenza; however, the use of health care services by high-risk adults was similar in the two groups. In the hospitalized cohort, RSV infection and influenza A resulted in similar lengths of stay, rates of use of intensive care (15 percent and 12 percent, respectively), and mortality (8 percent and 7 percent, respectively). On the basis of the diagnostic codes of the International Classification of Diseases, 9th Revision, Clinical Modification at discharge, RSV infection accounted for 10.6 percent of hospitalizations for pneumonia, 11.4 percent for chronic obstructive pulmonary disease, 5.4 percent for congestive heart failure, and 7.2 percent for asthma."*

RSV in the adult is rare, and may be becoming extinct. As part of global warming, the RSV season is shrinking in England. If it gets any warmer, RSV may become an organism of the past, like frogs and salamanders.

"The seasons associated with laboratory isolation of respiratory syncytial virus (RSV) (for 1981-2004) and RSV-related emergency department admissions (for 1990-2004) ended 3.1 and 2.5 weeks earlier, respectively, per 1 degrees C increase in annual cen-

tral England temperature (P=.002 and .043, respectively). Climate change may be shortening the RSV season."

See, global warming isn't so bad, now is it? Less RSV, more malaria, dengue and *Leishmania*. The future is so bright, I gotta wear shades.

Rationalization

Respiration. 2005 May-Jun;72(3):263-9. Respiratory syncytial virus pneumonitis in immunocompromised adults: clinical features and outcome. http://www.ncbi.nlm.nih.gov/pubmed/15942295

Clin Infect Dis. 2006 Mar 1;42(5):677-9. Epub 2006 Jan 25. Climate change and the end of the respiratory syncytial virus season. http://www.ncbi.nlm.nih.gov/pubmed/16447114

N Engl J Med. 2005 Apr 28;352(17):1749-59. Respiratory syncytial virus infection in elderly and high-risk adults. http://www.ncbi.nlm.nih.gov/pubmed/15858184

....

Follow the Bug

I ALWAYS follow the bug. Infections have patterns. Given a name for a bacterium, you can often predict both where it came from and where it is likely to go. It doesn't matter how unusual the infection might be, the bugs do not lie.

Today's patient had recently had a cryoablation of a kidney tumor. A cryoablation is exactly what it sounds like: they stick a probe through the back into the tumor and then crank down the temperature, turning the tumor into a snowball of dead adenocarcinoma.

Forty-eight hours later the patient spikes a fever and grows a gram negative rod in the blood, and it turns out to be a *Bacteroides fragilis*.

Hmmm. The treating physicians thought it was a complication of the ablation, a urosepsis, and treated the patient with antibiotics. The patient improved, then developed malaise and fevers a few weeks later that was culture negative but again responded to antibiotics. After the antibiotics finished, her symptoms relapsed and she was readmitted.

She had a leukocytosis and hematuria, but the rest of the exam was negative. No belly or flank pain, although there was still slight tenderness in the flank area. So they called me.

B. fragilis is NEVER is a cause of UTI/Kidney infection. Well, almost never. There are a smattering of cases, but a distinctly uncommon cause of a cystitis and bacteremia. It is an obligate anaerobe that is part of the normal colonic flora and is usually thought of as a harmless commensal. Only when it's displaced from its home after surgery or trauma can it cause infection, but then infections can be serious.

When I think *Bacteroides* I think something wrong with the bowel, and I figured that either the bowel done got froze or, like I see not infrequently, the dead tumor was seeded with *Bacteroides*. I see this when there is a liver tumor ablation, but the liver is directly downstream from the colon and its bacteria. The kidney isn't.

So I figured there had to be a hole in the colon and I ordered a CAT scan.

There was. A big collection of air and inflammation that was one with the colon, kidney and flank.

As best I can tell, this is not a reported complication of cryoablation of the kidney: I can find neither colonic injury nor anaerobic bacteremia on the PubMeds. You can get ice ball fractures, which can't be good.

The patient was eventually cured with surgery and antibiotics. Mostly surgery.

Always follow the bug; the bug never lies.

Rationalization

Int J Urol. 2004 Mar;11(3):133-41. Urinary tract and genito-urinary suppurative infections due to anaerobic bacteria. http://www.ncbi.nlm.nih.gov/pubmed/15009360

J Vasc Interv Radiol. 2010 Aug;21(8):1309-12. Ice ball fractures during percutaneous renal cryoablation: risk factors and potential implications. http://www.ncbi.nlm.nih.gov/pubmed/20619675

....

Clivus

THE patient is an elderly female who was seeing her primary care doctor for a week of a sore neck/throat. As an outpatient the exam was most unimpressive as were the labs, and no firm diagnosis was made.

About a week later the patient is admitted to the hospital with an altered mental status. A CT scan of the head shows pansinusitis and the lumbar puncture (spinal tap) has a protein of 250 (elevated), normal glucose, 150 white blood cells,, a mix of polymorphonuclear cells and monocytes. The presence of any white blood cells suggests a nervous system infection.

The next day the blood cultures grow first a gram positive rod then a gram positive cocci in chains. The former turns out to be *Clostridium perfringens* and the latter *Staphylococcus intermedius*. Hmm.

The physical exam is significant for nothing but the altered mental status. An MRI is done. The sphenoid sinus, which was chock full of fluid on the CT, is now empty—its back wall has vanished. There is a small C1-C2 epidural abscess as well as a retropharyngeal abscess in front of the clivus, or so said the radiology report.

I pause here to note I had no idea what the hell a "clivus" was. I know I knew once upon a time, as I did have to pass head and neck anatomy, almost 31 years ago. In the intervening years I had never heard the word clivus, except, perhaps, as an exclamation from Professor Frink of *The Simpsons*.

So there is a bone in the head called the clivus. To quote the Wikipedia for those of you with fading memories as well:

"The clivus (Latin for "slope") is a part of the cranium, a shallow depression behind the dorsum sellæ that slopes obliquely backward.

148

It forms a gradual sloping process at the anterior most portion of the basilar occipital bone at its junction with the sphenoid bone. On axial planes, it sits just posterior to the sphenoid sinuses. Just lateral to the clivus bilaterally is the foramen lacerum which contains the internal carotid artery, proximal to its anastamosis with the Circle of Willis. Posterior to the clivus is the basilar artery. The clivus supports the upper part of the pons."

There is a toilet and a wine with the same name. Unrelated products until too much of the latter leads to worship at the former. Clivus. I think I will soon forget it once the patient is discharged. Clivus.

Looks like the infection eroded through the back of the sinus, where it drained into the epidural and retropharyngeal space, and then the bacteremia. But why the week of neck pain if the erosion occurred after admission? I worried when it was just the *Clostridium* that it was a metastatic infection from a bowel cancer, but we found nothing of note in the bowel.

Eventually the patient went to the OR for debridement of the retropharyngeal abscess, which had partially spontaneously drained into the throat and grew pure culture *Candida albicans*.

This is both an odd collection of organisms, and an unusual manifestation of a sphenoid infection, most erosions occurring from pituitary tumors. There is a smattering of similar cases, but not many. A smattering is more than 1 but less than 13.

She is on antibiotics and improving and we are trying to decide how and when to fix the hole in the sinus. Clivus. I have remembered it this far.

In the end she did fine.

Rationalization

Otolaryngol Head Neck Surg. 2001 Jul;125(1):101-2. Sphenoid sinusitis caused by Clostridium perfringens.

Br J Neurosurg. 2007 Dec;21(6):616-8. Intracranial epidural abscess secondary to isolated sphenoid sinusitis. http://www.ncbi.nlm.nih.gov/pubmed/18071992

POLL RESULTS

In response to the MRI, I would say
- You should all listen to what i say.
- My I.Q. is 199 for crying out flayven 198...197... 20%
- HOYVIN-GLAVIN! 10%
- I first observed this technology at the airport gift shop. 15%
- "And the clavus and the sphenoid and the hey hey hey!" 30%
- You won't enjoy it on as many levels as I do... Mm-hai bw-ha whoa-hoa. The colours children. Mwa-ha-lee 20%

The Real Deal?

I s this the real deal?

Today's case is an elderly patient who is admitted with decreased mental status and who cannot protect his airway. He has new bilateral lower lobe consolidative infiltrates on chest x-ray and is admitted for pneumonia.

In the last three months he has received two courses of antibiotics for pneumonia, the first for community acquired and the second for hospital acquired. He is a diabetic and has received several recent courses of prednisone for asthma/chronic obstructive pulmonary disease

So he gets a bronchoscopy, which shows heavy growth of *Candida* in his lung. Is this *Candida* pneumonia? I usually tell the residents that you can cut off all my fingers and count the number of true *Candida* pulmonary infections I have seen on my thumbs.

One case was what was thought to be an *Aspergillus* fungus ball that was causing recurrent hemoptysis—but at resection was a glob of a wet papier mâché-like material that grew pure *Candida albicans*.

The other was a massive and fatal aspiration. At autopsy the lung alveoli were filled with *Candida* hyphae. As the ever-wise Infectious Disease Society of America would say:

"Growth of Candida from respiratory secretions rarely indicates invasive candidiasis and should not be treated with antifungal therapy...Candida pneumonia and lung abscess are very uncommon...Only rarely after aspiration of oropharyngeal material does a primary Candida pneumonia or abscess develop. Unfortunately, a positive culture from respiratory secretions is frequently used as an indication to initiate antifungal therapy in febrile patients who have no other evidence of invasive disease. Multiple prospective and retrospective studies, including autopsy studies, consistently demonstrate the poor predictive value of the growth of Candida from respiratory secretions, including bronchoalveolar lavage fluid. Because of the rarity of Candida pneumonia, the extremely common finding of Candida in respiratory secretions, and the lack of specificity of this finding, a decision to initiate antifungal therapy should not be made on the basis of respiratory tract culture results alone"

Not that anyone in the ICU can ignore a *Candida* in a bronchpscopy.

So I am skeptical that the *Candida* is the real deal, despite all the risk factors, especially when it is a *Candida glabrata*. *C. glabrata* pneumonia is extremely rare, so I figure, no way. And then.

The 1-beta-D-glucan, a test for *Candida*, comes back positive, at a little over 2x the lower limit. I am still unenthused, given the operational characteristics of the test, that the *Candida* is the cause of pneumonia, but given the all the co-morbidities, it is the tipping point. I treat. Grumble grumble.

The longer I am in medicine, the more I appreciate the indecision of Hamlet. Trying to make important decisions based on suspect information is not really like having to worry about whether to kill my stepfather, mind you. I just need decide on a course of therapy or not. But do not listen to me talk from behind the arras.

Rationalization

Clinical Practice Guidelines for the Management of Candidiasis:

2009 Update by the Infectious Diseases Society of America

http://cid.oxfordjournals.org/content/48/5/503.1.full.pdf+html

Intern Med. 2005 Nov;44(11):1191-4. A probable case of aspiration pneumonia caused by Candida glabrata in a non-neutropenic patient with candidemia. http://www.ncbi.nlm.nih.gov/pubmed/16357460

....

Unexpecting the Unexpected

THE patient had shoulder surgery after an injury a year ago. It gets infected at another hospital. The cultures grow *Propionibacterium acnes* and he has a course of antibiotics. Five months pass with no problems. No rubor, no dolor, no calor, no tumor. The shoulder is aspirated. Nothing. Inflammatory markers (erythrocycte sedimentation rate and C-reactive protein) are all normal. He is admitted for further arthroscopic repair work. At surgery, the joint and surrounding tissues are pristine and the repair is done.

Good news, I tell the patient, it looks like there is no sign of any infection. No need for any further antibiotics. Not a sign of a whiff of a suggestion of infection. To make sure, I have the cultures held for two weeks, and after a fortnight, the cultures are negative.

P. acnes is a not uncommon (nothing obscures like a double negative) anaerobic gram positive rod that lives in greasy hair follicles, which is why it is seen more often in males than in unfortunately furry females. It is probably a more common infection of prosthetic infections (joints and lines) than is suspected. If you really want to find the organism you have to hold the cultures for two weeks. Or have the lab hold it. No sense in filling your hands with cultures. It is, by the way, one of the few metronidazole-resistant anaerobes. The infections it causes are usually indolent, with months and years passing between the surgery and the clinical infection. It does not, as a rule, cause an acute infection.

I figure I will never hear from the patient again.

You know where this is going, don't you?

Four weeks after the surgery the patient is seen in follow-up with swelling at the anterior and posterior scope ports. I push on one and dark, slightly black/yellow thin fluid squirts out.

Early in my practice I was evaluating an infected port and I gave it a gentle push with my finger. That was when it decided to rupture, squirting pus up my tie and stopping just short of my slightly open mouth. This was in the era before widespread personal protective equipment, but I was not expecting the pus to shoot out like a super soaker. I now make sure any pus will directed towards my resident. Just kidding.

In the OR the surgeons find a diffuse white, granular, not classic, pus inside the shoulder. Gram stain is negative, but the cultures all grow, yep. *P acnes.*

What?!?!?!?!?!

New infection? Relapse? Where was it before? Why is it acute instead of an indolent infection? I do not get this case. It would have been a lot easier if the patient had read the textbook and presented more typically. Now it is another long course of antibiotics, this time clindamycin, but what to do next time when he needs further repairs?

Treat even if there are no signs and symptoms of infections, like I didn't do this time? Not be swayed by past experience? Argh. I hate the inordinate influence inflicted by cases that do not go as they should. I know there are always outliers, but you cannot let outliers dictate practice. Oh well, I have a few months to fret about it.

Rationalization

Propionobacter acnes Infection as an Occult Cause of Postoperative Shoulder Pain: A Case Series. Clin Orthop Relat Res. 2011 http://www.ncbi.nlm.nih.gov/pubmed/21240577

J Shoulder Elbow Surg. 2010 Mar;19(2):303-7. Epub 2009 Nov 1. Propionibacterium acnes infection after shoulder arthroplasty: a diagnostic challenge. http://www.ncbi.nlm.nih.gov/pubmed/19884021

POLL RESULTS

Unusual outcomes
* Never alter my practice. 0%
* Always alter my practice. 33%
* I never have unusual outcomes. 0%
* Practice makes mediocre. It's why its called practice. 29%
* Denial keeps me happy. It is more than a river in Syria. 38%

SHAZAM

TODAY's patient has a UTI. Nothing unusual—However, it is due to *Staphylococcus aureus*. *S. aureus* in a sterile site should always lead to two questions: where did it come from and where did it go?

S. aureus in the urine should give one pause, especially if it is in a male and not associated with prior instrumentation (by which I mean a Foley catheter or a trans-urethral resection of the prostate, not a flute or a tuba).

Staph in the urine can be due to hematogenous seeding. It is one of the few bugs in the urine that doesn't necessarily get there retrograde. Not every time, but you have to ask the question: was this hematogenous seeding?

"Even though UT catheterization is the main predisposing factor for primary SA UTI, some cases may be mediated through unrecognized preceding bacteremia related to intravascular device exposure or other healthcare-related factors."

S. aureus in the urine is a bad sign in those who are bacteremic.

"Among patients with S. aureus bacteremia, those with S. aureus bacteriuria had 3-fold higher mortality than those without bacteriuria, even after adjustment for comorbidities. Bacteriuria may identify patients with more severe bacteremia, who are at risk of worse outcomes."

Best I can tell, there is no reason for bacteremia or a UTI in this patient except for a large prostate, so you can guess that the patient is a male.

He also has severe back pain that is initially thought to be pyelonephritis, although signs of that are not seen on the CT scan. The pain was severe and he was bedbound from the severity, a 10/10.

So we got an MRI, and there was the discitis/epidural abscess you would expect. How did the Staph get there? Batson's venous plexus, of course. Or so I like to say.

You remember the Batson venous plexus? Not me. First time I had a case was late last century (and every case has been in males with a big prostate). I had to be "reminded" by Dr. Jones of its existence.

Let the Wikipedia be our guide:

"The Batson venous plexus, or Batson veins, is a network of valveless veins in the human body that connect the deep pelvic veins and thoracic veins (draining the inferior end of the urinary bladder, breast and prostate) to the internal vertebral venous plexuses...The plexus is named after anatomist Oscar Vivian Batson, who went on to become Captain Marvel...Batson's venous plexus may also allow the spread of infection in a similar manner. Urinary tract infections like pyelonephritis have been shown to spread to cause osteomyelitis of the vertebrae via this route."

I expect time and antibiotics will lead to resolution. So two pearls today. You can make a set of earrings.

Rationalization

Eur J Clin Microbiol Infect Dis. 2010 Sep;29(9):1095-101. Epub 2010 May 30.
Primary Staphylococcus aureus urinary tract infection: the role of undetected hematogenous seeding of the urinary tract. http://www.ncbi.nlm.nih.gov/pubmed/20703891

Staphylococcus aureus bacteriuria as a prognosticator for outcome of Staphylococcus aureus bacteremia: a case-control study BMC Infectious Diseases 2010, 10:225doi:10.1186/1471-2334-10-225

....

Life List

B EING an ID doc is like being a birdwatcher, although unlike birding, infectious diseases are actually interesting.

Like birding, I have mental list of all the infections and diseases I have yet to see. Like birds, some infections are rare and some are common. *Staphylococcus aureus* is a little brown bird. The HACEK group of organisms, causes of endocarditis, are rare. I have seen one of each (*Haemophilus* species [*Haemophilus parainfluenzae, Haemophilus aphrophilus, Haemophilus paraphrophilu*]), *Actinobacillus actinomycetemcomitans, Cardiobacterium hominis, Eikenella corrodens*, and *Kingella* species) in the last 24 years.

Unlike birders, I can't eat what I see. Well, I can. But *E coli* is not as tasty as Spotted Owl, which, if you are interested, is more flavorful than Ivory-Billed Woodpecker.

I had a little brown bird this week: *S. aureus* bacteremia with an epidural abscess. A common enough illness. But , as I have said before with *S. aureus*, you need to ask two questions. Where did it come from, and where did it go?

It came, I think, from his nose. The patient has daily nosebleeds from his Osler-Weber-Rendu disease. This is hereditary hemorrhagic telangiectasia, an autosomal dominant genetic disorder that causes development of abnormal blood vessels in the skin, mucous membranes, and internal organs, with associated bleeding. It is also called Rendu-Osler-Weber, and in some cases Weber is aced out entirely. It is also referred to as Babington's disease and Goldstein's haematemesis and Goldstein's syndrome. Who decides these names and their order, anyway? And what did Weber do to piss off the nomenclature mavens?

I digress.

Patients with hereditary telangiectasias are prone to get brain abscesses and lung abscesses, and a while back I discussed a patient who had recurrent *S. aureus* knee infections associated with hereditary telangiectasias. I never thought I would see a second case, so I put a check in my infectious disease life list.

I assume that he had a nosebleed and the staph gained access to the bloodstream from the nose and then to the epidural space.

"Among 353 patients with hereditary hemorrhagic telangiectasia retrospectively analyzed during the period 1985-2005, we identified 67 cases of severe infection that affected 48 patients (13.6%). Extracerebral infections accounted for 67% of all infections, and most involved Staphylococcus aureus and were associated with prolonged epistaxis. "

It was MSSA, not an uncommon finding in the nose:

"For 2001-2002, national S. aureus and MRSA colonization prevalence estimates were 32.4% (95% confidence interval [CI], 30.7%-34.1%) and 0.8% (95% CI, 0.4%-1.4%), respectively."

It is interesting that the MRSA rates were only 0.8%. In Vancouver, Washington, where the state mandates screening, we are running about 4%.

That's now two hereditary telangiectasias on my Life List, sort of a South Polar Skua in Oregon. Now the question is, do diseases, like celebrity deaths and Powerpuff Girls, come in threes?

Rationalization

Medicina (B Aires). 2007;67(6 Pt 2):714-6. [Spinal abscess in a patient with hereditary hemorrhagic telangiectasia]. http://www.ncbi. nlm.nih.gov/pubmed/18422064

J Infect Dis. 2006 Jan 15;193(2):172-9. Epub 2005 Dec 15.Prevalence of Staphylococcus aureus nasal colonization in the United States, 2001-2002. http://www.ncbi.nlm.nih.gov/pubmed/16362880

Clin Infect Dis. 2007 Mar 15;44(6):841-5. Epub 2007 Feb 1. Hemorrhagic hereditary telangiectasia (Rendu-Osler disease) and infectious diseases: an underestimated association. http://www.ncbi. nlm.nih.gov/pubmed?term=17304458

POLL RESULTS

I would prefer to add to my Life List
* a rare infection. 21%
* a rare bird. 21%
* a rare bird with a rare infection. Best of both worlds. 38%
* a rare disease that is not related to infections, and is not that interesting, but not everyone can be in ID. 13%
* click other and list the disease, bird, or other rarity of interest. Remember, rare, not mythical. 4%

Did Not See That Coming. Yet Again

Septic arthritis, or arth-a-ritis, is a common cause of consult. Often there is an obvious reason for the infection, like endocarditis or a recent joint space exploration by an orthopedic surgeon. This week, and today is only Wednesday, I have had four consults with septic joints and I have one for tomorrow. The joints are jumpin'.

The patient is in his 80s, demented and from a nursing home, and presents with a red, hot, swollen wrist. No other joint is involved and the rest of the history is apparently noncontributory. No reason to suspect seeding from another site; the nursing home records indicate fevers started the day the joint went bad.

Probably Staph, I said, maybe a Strep, like group G or B, not unusual for a spontaneous joint infection. In the OR there was a lot of pus in several of the joints of the wrist. Evidently the wrist has a bunch of bones and joints that can become infected. In my younger days, when I would bounce with a fall instead of break, I liked to rollerblade for exercise. I wore wrist protectors, much to the derision of my kids, to prevent a fracture of these unnamable bones. I remember in medical school memorizing all the bones in the wrist, and it was information that has yet to be relevant to my practice. And don't get me started on why I had to learn the difference between digoxin, digitoxin, and ouabain.

The blood and the joint have gram positive cocci in chains,

so a Strep, and I put him on penicillin and fret a little. He has a bioprosthesis where the aortic valve should be and, while there are no stigmata of endocarditis and a negative echocardiogram, I worry. Well, the name of the bug will make it all clear, right? Wrong.

Streptococcus pneumoniae. Didn't see that comin'.

How much should I worry about the valve? Both a lot and a little. There are a whopping two cases on the PubMeds of prosthetic valve endocarditis due to *S. pneumoniae,* and clinically he has nothing to suggest a third. Still...

Fortunately, the patient needs a course of IV antibiotics for the septic joint, and out of paranoia I will extend the therapy a few weeks extra. The MIC is quite low at 0.025, so I should be able to nuke it if it has settled on the valve.

The other issue is the patient's anion gap is zero. As an intern, back last century when gas was 93 cents a gallon, I had a patient with low anion gap and my resident pimped me on the reasons. I didn't know. The answer is a paraproteinemia, a proliferation of abnormal antibodies or fragments called "paraproteins." These paraproteins can indicate a hematological malignancy, either multiple myeloma or Waldenström's macroglobinema. My patient back in the day had Waldenström's. Paraproteinemias imply abnormal levels of normal, functioning antibodies that keep infections at bay, so they are also a reason for *S. pneumoniae* in the blood. I had a serum protein electrophoresis (SPEP) test done to look for a paraprotein.

The SPEP had one big peak representing a "monoclonal spike," showing the paraprotein of multiple myeloma.

Rationalization

Arch Intern Med. 1996 Oct 14;156(18):2141, 2146, 2148. Prosthetic valve endocarditis due to Streptococcus pneumoniae.

South Med J. 1998 Jul;91(7):624-9. Low anion gap. http://www.ncbi.nlm.nih.gov/pubmed/9671832

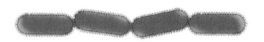

Mysteries

THE cases in this book are always chosen to make me look like the world's greatest diagnostician. Of course, that is usually the one case in five that has a firm answer. Most cases are a best guess, and there is no shortage of cases where I have to give a huge Gallic shrug and say, I don't know.

The big mystery case this week started with a week of feeling poorly, had severe left- sided pain, came to the ER. There was an enlarged, ruptured spleen and he was off to the OR for splenectomy.

Now on a ventilator for the last week, he has fevers, disseminated intravascular coagulation (DIC), pressor-dependent hypotension that resulted, eventually, in necrotic digits, an ongoing leukocytosis and marked left shift (immature white blood cells), anemia, and renal failure. He's finally slowly improving, but I do not know what he has. Pathology is negative. And I thought the pathologist always had the final say.

There is the infectious differential of splenic rupture: Epstein-Barr virus, malaria, *Babesia*, cytomegalovirus and the occasional abscess and parasite. He has none of the above.

There is the differential of sepsis with DIC and marked thrombosis, the purpura fulminans: Meningococcemia, *Capnocytophagia*, plague. He has none of these either, and there is no overlap on the Venn diagrams for the two processes.

Occasionally there is splenic rupture with polyarteritis nodosa and a smattering of other underlying pathologic processes.

Is this thrombotic thrombocytopenic purpura/ hemolytic-uremic syndrome (TTP/HUS)? He is hemolyzing, is thrombotic and thrombocytopenic, but has never had purpura, and there is only the occasional schistocyte on the peripheral smear. Schistocytes are broken remains of red cells fragmented by thrombin, and are <0.5% of red cells in normal people and slightly higher than that but still less than 1% in DIC. In cases of TTP/HUS there should be many more, 3-10%, not seen in this patient.

There are one or two cases of splenic rupture with HUS reported to be associated with Evans syndrome, a rare autoimmune disease that attacks but cells, but it is a weak association at best. Clinically he seems to be somewhere on the TTP/HUS continuum, but not firmly in either camp.

The patient is slowly improving, and once he's off the ventilator perhaps I can get a history that will lead to the diagnosis. But perhaps it just ruptured on its own. The spleen does that sometimes. Silly spleen.

Never did get a final, satisfying, diagnosis.

Rationalization

Med Clin (Barc). 2004 Oct 30;123(15):595-6. [Hemolytic-uremic syndrome secondary to acute pancreatitis with spontaneous spleen rupture].

Spontaneous Splenic Rupture Timothy Laseter; Tamara McReynolds Military Medicine, Volume 169, Number 8, August 2004, pp. 673-674(2).

EMERGENCY RADIOLOGY Volume 4, Number 6, 415-418 Spontaneous splenic rupture: Report of five cases and a review of the literature.

....

Toe Hold

THE patient is an elderly female who had a prosthetic valve placed two months ago at Outside Hospital.

Now the patient comes in SIRS-y. This is the systemic inflammatory response syndrome, a whole-body inflammation that is often (not always) associated with infection. She rapidly responds to antibiotics and all her blood cultures are growing a coagulase negative *Staphylococcus*. No surprise. Coagulase negative staphylococcus is a common cause of early (< 2 months post op) prosthetic valve endocarditis and can become symptomatic for up to a year after surgery. Transesophageal echocardiography is reassuringly negative for a ring abscess or a vegetation (infected clot on the valve), as best can be told.

There is no other reason by history and physical for multiple positive blood cultures for this organism. Then the lab identifies it as *S. lugdunensis*. What? I have written about this organism in the past: its preferred habitat is the big toe, it is a cause of lower extremity cellulitis and when found in the blood often means endocarditis.

"S. lugdunensis behaves more like S. aureus than other CNS in many respects, including exhibiting an elevated degree of virulence. S. lugdunensis is both a skin commensal and a pathogen responsible for nosocomial and community-acquired infections that may proceed aggressively and with a level of severity reminiscent of that of S. aureus infections."

It is rarely reported as a cause of prosthetic valve endocarditis, and I am surprised that a lower-body colonizer ended up as a probable valve infection, as the chest is a long way from the toe and the infection was presumptively acquired intraoperatively. The patient did not have saphenous vein grafting, just a valve replacement.

So how did the organism get to the valve, short of the patient being flexible enough to put a toe in her nose? It is hard to infect tissues hematogenously. Think IV heroin user. They inject bacteria daily, as does anyone who flosses and brushes, and seeding from this bacteremia is uncommon. The immune system takes care of the bacteria and they have no place to go. Bacteria do like clot, and in ID we frequently see infections in places with recent trauma. Presumably there is a little clot for the organism to settle on and cause infection.

Could the infection have been hematogenous? I do not know the practice at Outside Hospital, but there is not always respect given to scrubbing the hub of catheters before injecting medications and the hub could be a source for infection.

"The contaminated hands of anesthesia providers are a significant source of patient environmental and stopcock set contamination in the operating room. Intraoperative bacterial transmission to the IV stopcock set occurred in 11.5% (19/164) of cases, of which 47% (9/19) were of provider origin. Intraoperative bacterial transmission to the anesthesia environment occurred in 89% (146/164) of cases, 12% (17/146) of which were of provider origin."

I just imagine the anesthesiologist scratching her foot, then handling the line without a good hand or hub scrub, then, viola, foot-hand transfer and a touch of *S. lugdunensis* in the blood. Although this study looked at anesthesia—and far be it from me to cast aspersions on the infection control practices of my anesthesia colleagues across the country—it is probably widely applicable to all who access lines.

I will never know the source of the *S. lugdunensis*, although if I need a valve or a hip, I am going to hire someone to watch my case and remind everyone in the OR to scrub the hub.

Rationalization

Clin Microbiol Rev. 2008 Jan;21(1):111-33. From clinical microbiology to infection pathogenesis: how daring to be different works for Staphylococcus lugdunensis. http://www.ncbi.nlm.nih.gov/pmc/articles/PMC2223846/?tool=pubmed

Anesth Analg. 2011 Jan;112(1):98-105. Epub 2010 Aug 4. Hand contamination of anesthesia providers is an important risk factor for intraoperative bacterial transmission. http://www.ncbi.nlm.nih.gov/pubmed/20686007

Bayes-en At the Moon

THE last phone call of the day as I was leaving for a spring break vacation was a question about Lyme testing.

The questioner has a patient with weird neurologic symptoms, never been East of the Rockies, who went to a Naturopath, and they sent off a Lyme test and it was positive. So they did a spinal tap, and the IgM was indeterminate and the IgG negative. "What do you make of that?" they ask.

I want to say "You ordered the test, you interpret it." But I can't. I have to follow the 5 A's of being a consultant: affability, availability, ability, appearance, and accountability. Well, 4 out of 5 ain't bad.

There are two ways to get a Lyme serology, from your hospital lab and from private labs. Not all private labs offer tests that have been validated.

"CDC and the Food and Drug Administration (FDA) have become aware of commercial laboratories that conduct testing for Lyme disease by using assays whose accuracy and clinical usefulness have not been adequately established. These tests include urine antigen tests, immunofluorescent staining for cell wall—deficient forms of Borrelia burgdorferi, and lymphocyte transformation tests. In addition, some laboratories perform polymerase chain reaction tests for B. burgdorferi DNA on inappropriate specimens such as blood and urine or interpret Western blots using criteria that have not been validated and published in peer-reviewed scientific literature."

One of these labs, popular among Northwest naturopaths, was the one who'd done the diagnostic test on this patient. There was a blood smear for *Babesia* that they called positive. They gave a picture to the patient and I got a look at the smear, which had had an arrow pointing at a platelet clump. I was not impressed.

In this case it was an indeterminately, quasi-false positive.

IgM antibodies mark acute disease. CNS symptoms are late findings, so the test results in a patient with neurological complications of Lyme should be IgG positive, IgM negative. The serology does not match the clinical symptoms, which are not Lyme symptoms anyway.

But more importantly, if you order a test on a patient who does not have risks for disease and does not have symptoms of the disease, a positive test is extremely unlikely to be a true positive. So in this case the best you can do is generate anxiety and further testing working up a false positive.

Statistics makes my brain hurt. I took 4 years of math in college (physics major) but I took and dropped statistics 4 times, once a year for 4 years. Every time they got past the coin flipping they lost me. So far be it from me to pontificate about statistics, but still, I try and understand the concepts.

For testing it comes down to trying to internalize Bayes' Theorem, which I can't do. I tend to think Bayseanly when considering SCAMs (supplement, complementary and alternative medicine), where zero prior probability makes a positive study in, say homeopathy, extremely unlikely to be a true result.

For day-to=day applications of Bayes', there is an app for that. Rx-Bayes is a iOS app that allows you to alter the parameters of a test to determine its post-test probability. Odds are it is the best 99 cents you can spend on a medical app. Well, second best, after my app.

Even at a liberal 1% chance of disease, the post-test probability is only 14% (assuming a sensitivity of 85% and specificity of 95% for the test, a reasonable estimation from the literature).

It still makes my brain hurt, but is nice to fiddle with the sliders on Rx-Bayes when I am trying to determine what a test results will mean in terms of the probabilities that a patient actually has a disease.

I hope if I use it often enough I will actually understand Bayes' Theorem.

Ha.

Rationalization

Notice to Readers: Caution Regarding Testing for Lyme Disease http://www.cdc.gov/mmwr/preview/mmwrhtml/mm5405a6.htm

BetterExplained http://betterexplained.com/articles/an-intuitive-and-short-explanation-of-bayes-theorem/

An Intuitive Explanation of Bayes' Theorem http://yudkowsky.net/rational/bayes

Prior Probability: The Dirty Little Secret of "Evidence-Based Alternative Medicine" http://www.sciencebasedmedicine.org/?p=48

Rx-Bayes http://itunes.apple.com/us/app/rx-bayes/id413792280?mt=8&ign-mpt=uo%3D2

POLL RESULTS
Statistics
- I apply them daily to my practice. 17%
- I ain't never heard of no Bayes' Theorem. 8%
- I only use a p value in renal clinic. 10%
- Are a piece of cake. I am not one of the 5 out of 4 Americans who do not understand statistics. 23%
- Make my brain hurt as well. 33%
- Other Answers 8%
    1.   mmmm....cake
    2.   I am not a statistic. I am an anecdote.
    3.   are for people who don't already know everything

NSAIDs. Not Necessarily For What Ales You

THE "what" is simple enough: pneumococcal pneumonia with bacteremia. Not uncommon. The patient develops, however, one whopping empyema—pus in the chest cavity. Four large loculated collections of pus that require a video-assisted thorascopic surgery to drain.

The patient is relatively young, with no medical problems, so why such a huge empyema? No immunologic issues.

Inflammation is good and bad. It is good to have some inflammation, but too much inflammation may well kill the patient. The inflammatory response being a lot like beer: a little is good, a lot is bad.

I bet the reason that patients who get azithromycin as part of the community acquired pneumonia (CAP) therapy have a better outcome is not that you are treating atypical organisms, but that azithromycin takes the edge off the inflammatory response by suppressing pro-inflammatory cytokines.

"Three of the four tested macrolides, azithromycin, clarithromycin and roxithromycin, exhibited pronounced, concentration-related reduction of IL-1β, IL-6, IL-10, TNF-α, CCL3, CCL5, CCL20, CCL22, CXCL1, CXCL5, and G-CSF release. Further slight inhibitory effects on IL-1α, CXCL8, GM-CSF, and PAI-1 production were also observed."

But not FBI, CIA, LOL, OMG, or LSMFT.

That is one of many studies that demonstrate similar immunomodulation. Macrolides are a two-drink maximum at the pneumonia bar.

However, there are other ways to affect the inflammatory response in pneumonia. You can give steroids for CAP, an intervention still fraught with uncertainty. As the Cochrane review sums it up:

"In most patients with pneumonia, corticosteroids are generally beneficial for accelerating the time to resolution of symptoms. However, evidence from the included studies was not strong enough to make any recommendations."

Those who read my science-based medicine blog know I am not a fan of Cochrane, whose basic methodology is collecting multiple cow pies into one big pile and thinking the result is gold. Still, I like to quote the Cochrane when it confirms my pre-existing bias, and ignore it when it doesn't.

And then there are NSAIDs. NSAIDs are evil. Well, not evil, I am a big fan after an excessive weekend. But there is this ongoing suspicion that in some patients NSAIDs tip the balance in favor of the bacteria, leading to worser (a term my children used when young, and I have not abandoned) illness, not confirmed, but I am still suspicious:

"Case reports and retrospective studies suggest that the application of NSAIDs to relieve these nonspecific symptoms can delay diagnosis and treatment of GAS necrotizing fasciitis. However, prospective studies do not support a risk of developing GAS necrotizing fasciitis as a result of NSAID therapy, or a worsening of established streptococcal infection."

It is of interest the patient was on ibuprofen during the week of the illness and developed the empyema.

"Of the 90 patients included, 32 (36%) had taken NSAIDs prior to hospital referral. Compared with non exposed patients, they were younger and had fewer comorbidities but similar severity of disease at presentation, despite a longer duration of symptoms before referral. However, they more often developed pleuropulmonary complications, such as pleural empyema and lung cavitation (37.5% vs 7%; P = .0009), and had a trend to more-invasive disease, with a higher frequency of pleural empyema (25% vs 5%, P = .014) and bacteremia."

So maybe it was the ibuprofen. Or maybe not. Each of these drugs has a different effect on the inflammatory response, some good and some bad. I am a big fan of the inflammatory response, at least in the outpatient setting. Fevers are good, inflammation is good. It is why I do not put ibuprofen in my beer.

Rationalization

Pharmacol Res. 2011 Feb 17. [Epub ahead of print] Macrolide antibiotics broadly and distinctively inhibit cytokine and chemokine production by COPD sputum cells in vitro. http://www.ncbi.nlm.nih.gov/pubmed/21315154

Cochrane Database Syst Rev. 2011 Mar 16;3:CD007720. Corticosteroids for pneumonia. http://www.ncbi.nlm.nih.gov/pubmed/21412908

Medicine (Baltimore). 2003 Jul;82(4):225-35. Assessing the relationship between the use of nonsteroidal antiinflammatory drugs and necrotizing fasciitis caused by group A streptococcus http://www.ncbi.nlm.nih.gov/pubmed/12861100

Chest. 2011 Feb;139(2):387-94. Epub 2010 Aug 19. Nonsteroidal antiinflammatory drugs may affect the presentation and course of community-acquired pneumonia. http://www.ncbi.nlm.nih.gov/pubmed/20724739

POLL RESULTS
For me it's
- a Bud. 3%
- a Coors light aka tap water 14%
- Duff. 17%
- Billy Beer. Anyone remember Billy Beer? 7%
- Any beer from Oregon. 17%
- Other Answers 41%
    1. any real ale from the UK
    2. no beer!
    3. Microbrew or Fat Tire
    4. Sam Adams
    5. Guiness!
    6. Yuengling
    7. Turtle Anarchy! Of course we remember Billy Beer
    8. Alcohol is a tool of the devil

....

Delayed Disease

D ISEASES can be delayed.

I took care of a patient a month ago for meningitis. Off antibiotics for a month, he has the sudden onset of fevers and headache and comes to the ER. After admission, he develops three very loose stools and some mild abdominal pain. His white blood cell count is 12,000 per microliter, seriously elevated. It also has 30% band neutrophils, immature neutrophils indicating that the bone marrow has been stimulated to produce more white cells. But the lumbar puncture is negative.

The other is an elderly male who two months ago had a gastric perforation following a dilatation, and subsequently has had abdominal abscesses and a long antibiotic course after they are drained.. He too has been for home for about 6 weeks. He also presents with fevers, nausea, vomiting and then diarrhea. A complete blood count is normal.

Both are positive for *Clostridium difficile.*

Now I know that *C. difficile* can occur weeks after cessation of antibiotics. As I think about it, it annoys me to blame the antibiotics. Or should it?

I think of *C. difficile* like blackberry bushes that grow when you remove the normal foliage. That is the metaphor I use with patients. Supposedly the patient is a carrier:

" 94 (7.6%) individuals were positive for C. difficile by faecal culture but carriage rates among the study groups ranged from 4.2% to 15.3%. "

Antibiotics beat back the other flora and the *C. difficile* takes over. So why the delay of weeks? You would think that if *C. difficile* were there it would have taken over right away.

I suspect that the antibiotics did mess up the flora; studies suggest that effects of antibiotics on the GI flora last for months. An interesting question is which of the normal bacterial flora are most important in controlling *C. difficile?* And how long does it take to these organisms to be reconstituted? If that information is out there, I can't find it. It would make stool transplants simpler.

So my patients have a messed up flora from antibiotics and then eat the wrong food (*C. diffiicle* is in the food we eat), get a new strain of *C. diffiicle*, and then a delayed diarrhea. The source of the infection is not the hospital but the diet. We just tilled the soil.

Any why the nausea and vomiting in a colonic bug? Is toxin leaking into the blood stream (probably) to cause central nausea and vomiting? Or does eating *C. difficile* lead to upper GI symptoms due to toxin production in the stomach and small bowel, before heading (anus-ing?) down the bowel to the colon?

Far more questions today than answers. That's medicine. I often feel I know less and less about more and more and some day I will know nothing about everything. At least I have the Web.

Rationalization

J Med Microbiol. 2001 Aug;50(8):720-7. Colonisation and transmission of Clostridium difficile in healthy individuals examined by PCR ribotyping and pulsed-field gel electrophoresis. http://www.ncbi.nlm.nih.gov/pubmed/11478676

J Chemother. 1990 Aug;2(4):218-37. Impact of antimicrobial agents on human intestinal microflora. http://www.ncbi.nlm.nih.gov/pubmed/2230905

Clin Infect Dis. 2010 Sep 1;51(5):577-82. Clostridium difficile in food and domestic animals: a new foodborne pathogen? http://www.ncbi.nlm.nih.gov/pubmed/20642351

POLL RESULTS
As for me
- I know everything I need to know. 2%
- The more I learn, the less I know. 63%

- With Google and Pubmed, who needs to know anything? 17%
- I scoff at your reality-based approach; I do not need facts, I prefer opinions. 8%
- If it feels right, it must be true. 6%
- Other Answers 4%
    1. I've had C. diff, and I empathize
    2. the more i learn, the more I know. but also realize that incompleteness of our understanding of things.

Playing From the Tips

D ID you hear about the urologist who did not charge for circumcision? He just took tips.

So I get lots of curbsides: questions of interest to the calling doctor, and often I do not have good answers.

About two weeks ago I got a call. A patient is going home after being admitted with a fever. He had an indwelling intravenous catheter used for total parenteral nutrition for short bowel syndrome. The line was pulled in case it was a cause of the fever, and blood cultures are negative, but the line tip is growing greater than 15 colonies of *Candida albicans*. I had moved on (I cover three hospitals) and the patient is to be out the door in mere moments.

What to do?

Good question. What should you do with a positive catheter tip and negative blood cultures?

"Eight (2.6%; 95% CI 1.2-5.1) of the 312 patients yielding isolated bacterial or fungal CVC tip cultures (with negative blood cultures) developed subsequent bloodstream infection (BSI) caused by the same species as that isolated from the tip culture (Staphylococcus aureus, 1: Enterococcus spp.; 2: Pseudomonas aeruginosa; and 3: Candida spp.)."

So it is a risk, but a small one, for future bloodstream infections, and it may be of more importance for patients on TPN, especially if the patient remains febrile after pulling the line, which this patient did not. *S. aureus* on a line tip with negative blood cultures should probably get a course of an undecided antibiotic for an unknown duration, but *Candida?*

So I suggested fluconazole, which the patient received in a new line placed on the other side. The patient has no peripheral access (bad veins) and is dependent on IV fluids, so a new central line had been placed.

Seven days later, the fevers are back, and this time the blood grows *C. albicans* as does the catheter tip. Again.

The heck. And the CT shows peripheral lung nodules that are classic for septic emboli.

Has to be right-sided endocarditis, right? Even though the repeat blood cultures are negative and the patient's fever resolves right away. I bet the hospitalist 50 cents (I am an ID doc, after all) that the transesophageal echocardiogram or the ultrasound of the great vessels would show clot.

Nope.

I also assume the yeast must be resistant to fluconazole (results take so long to return, I didn't bother to send the organism for testing), so it is a long course of caspofungin. And I still fret about the valve.

In the end the patient did fine with no third relapse of his fungemia.

Typical straightforward case.

Rationalization

Clin Microbiol Infect. 2010 Jun;16(6):742-6. Epub 2009 Sep 11. Development of bacteriemia or fungemia after removal of colonized central venous catheters in patients with negative concomitant blood cultures. http://www.ncbi.nlm.nih.gov/pubmed/19747217

J Hosp Infect. 2010 Oct;76(2):119-23. Epub 2010 Jun 16. Diagnosis of catheter-related bloodstream infection in a total parenteral nutrition population: inclusion of sepsis defervescence after removal of culture-positive central venous catheter. http://www.ncbi.nlm.nih.gov/pubmed/20554348

Clin Microbiol Infect. 2006 Sep;12(9):933-6. Clinical significance of isolated Staphylococcus aureus central venous catheter tip cultures. http://www.ncbi.nlm.nih.gov/pubmed/16882304

3640 Days Later

I ONCE made the mistake of watching the movie *28 Days Later*. The mistake was starting to watch the movie at 11 pm, on the computer, with headphones. I did not sleep that night.

Time passes, and bad things can happen when time passes. For those youngsters out there, just wait until you are in your 50s.

Twenty years ago the patient has a hip replaced. 10 years ago it is revised. Time passes.

Pain begins in the hip and increases. Slowly, but surely, the hip becomes more painful with use. No fevers, chills or other constitutional symptoms.

Plain x-ray films show a lot of heterotopic bone and a tap of the joint is done. No white blood cells in the tap, and one colony of *P. acnes* grows from a culture. Inflammatory markers, ESR and CRAP (C Re-Active Protein), are normal. Everything looks like the *P. acnes* is a contaminant, but this organism makes me nervous. It's a slow, shambling zombie, not the Rage virus variety, so I hedge.

The patient is taken to the OR for another revision.

Intraoperatively there is no purulence, some areas of bone lysis and other areas of heterotopic bone. Gram stain shows no organisms and no white blood cells.

Well, I tell the patient, looks like the you do not have an infection, but the cultures are the final arbitrator. I asked the lab to hold the cultures for two weeks, but after 5 days the cultures were growing *P. acnes*. Yet again, my clinical acumen dissed by the cultures.

P. acnes is an odd bug. It can fester for years before becoming evident. Fester. There is a word we do not use enough. It wasn't until I was a fellow that I recognized the significance of the name

Uncle Fester from the Addams Family.

"Fifty patients with prosthetic hip (34), knee (10) or shoulder (6) infections were included and analyzed according to their symptom-free interval: < or = 2 years for 35 and > 2 years for 15 (mean interval: 11+/-6 years). The numbers of previous prostheses (p=0.04) were higher for the shorter-interval group, which had more frequent signs of infection (p=0.004). These findings suggest infection in most of the patients whose PJI symptoms appeared: < or = 2 years after the index operation, and colonization in the majority of those whose symptoms appeared > 2 years after index surgery...

CONCLUSION: P. acnes can cause different types of PJI: late chronic infections, colonization of loosened prostheses and, exceptionally, acute postoperative infections."

Also, *P. acnes* does not incite much of an inflammatory response, perhaps because it has evolved to be a commensal. It has become so intimate with humans that the immune system mostly ignores it. No pus, no inflammation is often the case:

"Low-grade infection was systematically searched for in all revision shoulder surgeries by harvesting tissue samples. Ten consecutive patients were identified with a non-purulent low-grade infection of the shoulder. All of these patients suffered from pain and eight were stiff. Preoperative aspiration in eight patients yielded bacterial growth in only one case. Serum C-reactive protein levels were normal in seven out of 10 cases. Propionibacterium acnes was identified in seven..."

Since it resides in hair follicles living on fatty acids in the sebaceous glands and on sebum secreted by follicles, it is protected from both the prophylactic antibiotics and the topical antiseptics. And it has to have the worst diet of any bacteria outside the colon. It is also one of the few anaerobes that is resistant to metronidazole.

So a long course of clindamycin and I hope I get rid of the beast.

Rationalization

Chir Organi Mov. 2009 Apr;93 Suppl 1:S71-7. Non-purulent low-grade infection as cause of pain following shoulder surgery: preliminary results. http://www.ncbi.nlm.nih.gov/pubmed/19711173

J Infect. 2007 Aug;55(2):119-24. Epub 2007 Apr 5. Propionibacterium acnes: an agent of prosthetic joint infection and colonization. http://www.ncbi.nlm.nih.gov/pubmed/17418419

POLL RESULTS

I most resemble
- Uncle Fester 24%
- Cousin Itt 32%
- Pugsly 12%
- Gomez 8%
- Lurch 16%
- Other Answers 8%
  1. lon chaney
  2. Wednesday

Creative Diagnostic Modalities

I WORK in a good environment. I spend 95% of my clinical time in the hospital, and those who work in hospitals tend to be of high caliber. The worst I can say about a few of my colleagues is they are competent; the rest are excellent. There is a distinct lack of people I would consider poor at what they do. As a result, it is rare to get a "dumb" consult.

Not so true in the outpatient setting. I get the occasional patient who has a diagnosis by a naturopath—and let's be generous, shall we, and say that these diagnoses are made in very, well, creative ways. It may be confirmation bias, but I have yet to see a legitimate diagnosis by a naturopath. Infectious diseases, or medicine, are not their strong suit, I suppose.

I recently saw a patient who had unexplained abdominal pain for a year and a half. The patient had an extensive evaluation and no explanation for the symptoms, and eventually wandered into the arms of a naturopath looking for answers.

Now mind you, the patient did not have symptoms that could be reasonably ascribed to parasites or worms, and, more importantly, had no risks for parasites or worms. The industrialized West is reasonably free of worms and their brethren. The naturopath did not do serology or blood work or even a simple stool study looking for the eggs of various worms. It is how I, along with a history and physical looking for the pattern of disease that marks a parasite, make a diagnosis.

No, he or she (I do not remember the pronoun used at the time) proudly used electrodiagnosis. Proudly. As my patient related it to me, the naturopath, a graduate of Bastyr, considered him/herself to be an expert in parasite treatment and diagnosis.

What is electrodiagnosis, you ask?

There are many electrodiagnostic devices out there, so I do not know precisely which one the ND used. It was described as follows: the patient held an electrode one hand, the naturopathic expert in parasitology touched another probe to various positions on the body, twirled a dial, and announced that the reading indicated parasites. Really. I am proud that I did not burst out laughing during the interview, as from my perspective the diagnosis was a joke.

Electrodiagnosis is said to measure disturbances in the body's flow of "electro-magnetic energy" along "acupuncture meridians" but are usually only galvanometers that measure electrical resistance of the patients' skin. The technique is sometimes called electroacupuncture or EAV. It was—invented? discovered? pulled out of Dr Voll's imagination, yeah, that's it, imagination?—in the 1950's:

"The basic concept for all of the ElectroDermal screening devices, was the invention of Dr. Reinhardt Voll, who in the 1940s, discovered that the electrical resistance of the human body is not homogenous and that meridians existed over the body which may be demonstrated as electrical fields. Furthermore, he showed that the skin is a semi-insulator to the outside environment. By the

1950s Voll had learned that the body had at least 1000 points on the skin which followed the 12 lines of the classical Chinese meridians. Each of these points, Voll called a Measurement Point (MP). Working with an engineer, Fritz Werner, Voll created an instrument to measure the skin resistance at each of the acupuncture points, patterned after a technique called Galvanic Skin Resistance (GSR). This was named Point Testing. In 1953, Voll had established the procedure that became known as Electro-Acupuncture according to Voll (EAVJ)."

There is zero validity to making any diagnosis this way. Except, of course, the E-meter. E-meter forever. But those other electronic diagnostic devices? Pure bunkum. There is nothin' on the PubMeds on the validity of electrodiagnosis, and, on basic principles and prior probability, no reason to suspect that electrodiagnosis would have any utility in diagnosing parasites, or anything else. I could not say it better than Quackwatch:

"The devices are used to diagnose nonexistent health problems, select inappropriate treatment, and defraud insurance companies. The practitioners who use them are either delusional, dishonest, or both."

Despite this, my patient received prolonged courses of mebendazole, thiabendazole and praziquantel, all at half doses. Uncertain of which parasite to kill, the naturopath tried to kill them all. Good thing, come to think of it, that he did not use his infernal contraption to diagnose cancer; who knows how many anticancer medications would have been prescribed.

In the end the patient spent considerable amounts of money and took unneeded medications for an imaginary diagnosis.

The etiology of the pain? Got me. It is not due to an infection, that much I am reasonably certain, and once I wander outside of infections, I recognize my limitations.

POLL RESULTS

The most creative diagnostic modality I have seen is

- electrodiagnosis. 3%

- live blood analysis. 16%
- blocked qi judged by looking at the tongue. 32%
- applied kinesiology. 16%
- lyme testing done at ... well, the US has 30 f the worlds lawyers, and I am but a poor doctor. But you know. 23%
- Other Answers 10%
    1. Analysis of the irises
    2. aura sensing/adjustment

Kind of a Repeat

THIS is my third volume of case histories, all collected from blog posts written more or less every other day from September 2008 to April 2011. Amazingly, there is little repetition in the clinical material I present. ID is that amazing. The jokes, so called, maybe not so much. My humor, not so amazing.

I have three great cases, or maybe-great cases, cooking at the moment. Depending on the results of pending studies, I may wow you, but at the moment, things are more on the mundane side. Staph, staph and staph. If any bug pays my mortgage, it is staph.

The patient is a diabetic dialysis patient who twists his knee, then gets bacteremic from his dialysis catheter and the knee is seeded. It is MSSA and the knee is washed out and he's sent home on a course of vancomycin. It is convenient to give vancomycin, which is dosed once a week, but is it wise?

Vancomycin is, if anything, an archetype for a lousy piece of garbage antibiotic that stinks on ice—those are adjectives that can be applied to antibiotics, not "strong" or "powerful." Bacteriostatic rather than bactericidal with poor penetration into tissues, when compared to a beta-lactam (penicillin is a beta-lactam), vancomycin is demonstrably worse for MSSA.

For example

"...vancomycin treatment was associated with SAB-related mortality when independent predictors for SAB-related mortality and propensity score were considered (adjusted odds ratio of 3.3, 95%

confidence interval of 1.2 to 9.5). In the case–control study using the objective matching scoring system and the propensity score system, SAB-related mortality in case patients was 37% (10/27) and in control patients 11% (6/54) (P < 0.01). Our data suggest that vancomycin is inferior to beta-lactam in the treatment of MSSA-B."

and

"Treatment failure was more common among patients receiving vancomycin (31.2% vs. 13%; P = .02). In the multivariable analysis, factors independently associated with treatment failure included vancomycin use (odds ratio, 3.53; 95% confidence interval, 1.15 13.45) and retention of the hemodialysis access (odds ratio, 4.99; 95% confidence interval, 1.89 13.76). Conclusions. Hemodialysis-dependent patients with MSSA bacteremia treated with vancomycin are at a higher risk of experiencing treatment failure than are those receiving cefazolin."

After the patient finished the vancomycin, the knee infection relapsed. Cefazolin can be easily dosed with dialysis as well: 1 gram after dialysis if 24 hours between runs, 2 grams if 48 and 3 grams if 72.

The take-home message? ALWAYS use a beta-lactam for *S. aureus* if you can. It is better than any other antibiotic we have.

And don't give strong, or powerful, or big gun, give appropriate antibiotics: the one that kills the bug in the space that is infected.

Rationalization

Antimicrob Agents Chemother. 2008 Jan;52(1):192-7. Epub 2007 Nov 5. Outcome of vancomycin treatment in patients with methicillin-susceptible Staphylococcus aureus bacteremia. http://www.ncbi.nlm.nih.gov/pubmed/17984229

Clin Infect Dis. 2007 Jan 15;44(2):190-6. Epub 2006 Dec 8. Use of vancomycin or first-generation cephalosporins for the treatment of hemodialysis-dependent patients with methicillin-susceptible Staphylococcus aureus bacteremia. http://www.ncbi.nlm.nih.gov/pubmed/17173215

POLL RESULTS

May favorite description for antibiotics is

- strong, big gun, powerful. Up yours, Crislip. 5%
- overpriced and overused 41%
- whatever the rep tells me is what I think. 11%
- the only true miracle drug in the medical armamentarium. Isn't that a glass container for growing armaments? 19%
- better than Old Spice. 19%
- Other Answers 5%
  1. Food
  2. A lifesaver. Without antibiotics I would be dead.

Dead Men Tell No Wives

IT is not uncommon when I ask a patient why they are in the hospital they say, in a surly voice, something like "my wife made me come" or "my girlfriend made me come." I think if it wasn't for the female half of the species most men would've died in their mid-20s of some treatable disease or other.

Such as with this case. An elderly man has had three weeks of progressive decline. He has had fevers, malaise and decreasing energy. He was barely able to accomplish his activities of daily living but toughed it out, as men are wont to do. One day he fell off the toilet and could not get back up. His wife brought him in as he was too ill to refuse.

The patient has known valvular heart disease, and for the last two months had ongoing issues with dental abscesses for which he was seeking care.

They get blood cultures in the emergency room. These turn positive and the lab tells me it's cascading gram-positive rods. Huh! Maybe it's some sort of *Corynebacterium*. It would be distinctly unusual to get this organism as a cause of endocarditis, but my career is based on people getting distinctly unusual organisms infecting them for no good reason. So I started vancomycin and and ampicillin as I don't want to miss *Listeria*. Gram-positive rods, and *Listeria*, have fooled me in the past. As the old saying goes, fool me once, shame on [pauses] shame on you. Fool me twice [pauses] You can't get fooled again.

And wouldn't you know it, the organism didn't read the textbook. It's a *Streptococcus*. Typical viridans group that causes endocarditis in the elderly. The lab tells me that sometimes on the plates a *Streptococcus* will look like small gram-positive rods.

In my practice, of course, endocarditis is not an unusual diagnosis. I see maybe a case a month. For me it's a relatively common diagnosis. In the general community most docs may see one or two a career.

More importantly, however, is fever in the elderly. If someone is older than age 55, and they have a fever, it probably represents a serious underlying medical problem. The cause of fevers in the young is usually trivial but fever in the elderly is usually serious.

I learned this as an intern griping about a patient being admitted for fever that had no obvious reason. The patient was elderly and as I pushed the gurney to her room (it was a county hospital; we often served as orderlies as well as blood draw technicians) she went into septic shock and almost died. The next day her blood cultures grew an enterococcus if memory serves me well. I didn't think she looked all that sick except for the fever. I guess that's why we do internships. So we gain some experience and we don't make mistakes when we are on our own.

Anyway, if you look in the literature you find that if you're elderly and present to the ER with a fever you have a real chance of having something seriously wrong.

"To study the effect of age on ultimate outcome of febrile illness, the authors prospectively studied 1,202 adult patients who came to an emergency room/walk-in clinic setting with temperatures of 101.0 degrees F (38.3 degrees C) or more. The patients were divided into four age categories: 17 to 40 years, 40 to 59 years, 60 to 79 years, and 80 years old or older. Advancing age was significantly (P less than 0.0005) associated with more serious disease, a higher rate of bacterial pathogen isolation, and a higher rate of life-threatening or deadly consequences. Of patients 17–39 years old, 58.2 per cent had viral syndromes, otitis media, or pharyngi-

tis as the causes of fever. Of patients aged 40-59 years, only 20.7 per cent had one of these diseases. However, of patients 60 years old or older, only 4.1 per cent (15 of 370) had viral syndromes, otitis media, or pharyngitis, and the overall rate of hospitalization for this group was 92.5 per cent. The authors conclude that febrile patients 60 years old or older seen in emergency room/ambulatory care settings are extremely likely to have serious diseases. Caution should be exercised before concluding that their fevers are of benign origin."

and

"Of the 470 patients with complete follow-up data, 357 (76.0%) had indicators of serious illness. Clinical features found to be independently associated with serious illness included oral temperature of 103 degrees F (39.4 degrees C) or more, respiration rate of 30 or more, leukocytosis of 11.0 x 10(9)/L or more, presence of an infiltrate, and pulse of 120 or more. At least one indicator of serious illness was present in 63 of 128 patients (49.6%) with none of these independently predictive clinical features. The most common final diagnoses were pneumonia (24.0%), urinary-tract infection (21.7%), and sepsis (12.8%).

CONCLUSION: Fever among geriatric ED patients frequently marks the presence of serious illness. All such patients should be strongly considered for hospital admission, particularly when certain clinical features are present. The absence of abnormal findings does not reliably rule out the possibility of serious illness."

I remain skeptical that the procalcitonin is a good way to help weed out who does and does not have bacterial infection, at least an emergency room. Others seem to swear by the test. I'm more likely to swear at the test. And its sensitivity and specificity are not that good. At least not good enough to bet someone's life on it.

"Among 243 patients included in the study, 167 had bacterial/parasitic infections, 35 had viral infections and 41 had other diagnoses. The PCT assay, with a 0.2 microg/l cutoff value, had a sensitivity of 0.77 and a specificity of 0.59 in diagnosing bac-

*terial/parasitic infection. Of the patients with PCT 5 microg/l
or greater, 51% had critical illness (death or intensive care unit
admission) as compared with 13% of patients with lower PCT
values.*"

If it is an old man (and that old man might be me) presenting
with a fever—or for that matter any man—it's probably been fes-
tering for a long time. If it wasn't for their female partner they'd
probably be dead. Despite that, I always get the distinct impres-
sion that the male of the twosome resents the meddling of his
spouse or girlfriend. Most men, I think, would rather be dead
than shown to be wrong. Good thing I am never wrong.

Rationalization

J Am Geriatr Soc. 1984 Apr;32(4):282-7. Effect of aging on the clinical significance of fever in ambulatory adult patients. http://www.ncbi.
nlm.nih.gov/pubmed/6707408

Ann Emerg Med. 1995 Jul;26(1):18-24. Fever in geriatric emergency
patients: clinical features associated with serious illness. http://www.
ncbi.nlm.nih.gov/pubmed/7793715

Crit Care. 2007;11(3):R60. Serum procalcitonin measurement as
diagnostic and prognostic marker in febrile adult patients presenting to the emergency department. http://www.ncbi.nlm.nih.gov/
pubmed/17521430

POLL RESULTS

I'm male and
- don't worry about fevers. 3%
- don't worry about chest pain. 13%
- don't worry about shortness of breath. 7%
- don't worry about fainting. 0%
- don't worry about a long life. 57%
- Other Answers 20%
    1. Do or do not, there is no worry.
    2. female at the same time
    3. not male; but don't nag my spouse, as he runs to MDs
    4. I am female

What To Do, What To Do

THE patient has a mitral valve repair. The middle, redundant part of the posterior leaflet is resected, making a wedge-shaped defect, then the remaining parts are sewn back together. To make sure the heart doesn't stretch and rip the repair asunder, a ring is sewn into the atrium to stabilize the valve.

To make it more tricky, it is done with robotic surgery, which I imagine being done by the robot from *Lost In Space*, waving his arms and shouting "Danger, Danger" whenever there is a break in sterile technique. Or maybe that's just me and wishful thinking.

The patient does well for the first week after discharge, then develops fevers and is admitted. All the blood cultures grow MSSA, and, no surprise, transthoracic echocardiography (TTE) is negative.

Who trusts a TTE for endocarditis? Not me.

We get a transesophageal (TEE) and there is a 1 cm vegetation on the valve, but the ring looks good.

The literature suggests that a mitral valve repair has about a 1% endocarditis rate, about the same as a valve replacement, but with better overall functional results.

What to do?

It is not really prosthetic valve endocarditis, but not native valve either, since the vegetation probably sits right on the suture line of the valve. At least the ring appears to be uninvolved. For MSSA prosthetic valve endocarditis, early surgery is probably the way to go. In this case? No literature to guide me. There are only reports of endocarditis in series in the surgical literature and they mention the endocarditis in passing. You know, the infection was not that interesting compared to the hemodynamic results. How the endocarditis was treated and whether medical therapy alone was effective, I cannot find with my PubMed or Google-Fu.

I plan on treating like prosthetic valve endocarditis with nafcillin, rifampin, and a two-week course of gentamicin, since the Gore-Tex sutures are probably infected—although I suppose they let the perspiration out of the vegetation and prevent the rain from getting in. We are big on Gore-Tex here in the perpetually rainy Pacific Northwest. And listening every day for the new murmur that heralds a tearing suture line.

It was a cure. Go, antibiotics. I'll miss them when they are gone.

Rationalization

European Journal of Cardio-Thoracic Surgery, Vol 9, 621-626. Improved results with mitral valve repair using new surgical techniques. http://ejcts.ctsnetjournals.org/cgi/content/abstract/9/11/621

Superiority of mitral valve repair in surgery for degenerative mitral regurgitation. Lee EM, Shapiro LM, Wells FC. Eur Heart J. 1997 Apr;18(4):655-63. http://www.ncbi.nlm.nih.gov/pubmed/9129898

POLL RESULTS

I would want Robot surgery by
- Tom Servo 25%
- Bender 17%
- Buffybot. 11%
- Gort 11%
- Marvin 22%
- Other Answers 14%
  1. Tobor
  2. R2D2
  3. R. Daneel Olivaw

....

Right the First Time

THE patient is a middle-aged male who initially came in with abdominal pain. A CAT scan showed he had ruptured his spleen. After his spleen was removed he became septic, but no diagnosis was ever made for the sepsis or a reason found for why the spleen ruptured. There are a smattering of cases in the literature of splenic rupture for no damn good reason; I suppose he fell into that category.

After a long and complicated ICU course he was moved to the floor. He then developed fevers and an increasing white blood cell count, and a fever workup ensued. The only thing that was found was a large area of fluid in the region of his former spleen that appeared to be old hematoma. Now since he was in recovering renal failure, the CAT scan was done without contrast agents, which can stress the kidneys. We could not tell whether or not there was an abscess in the area, and since there was no other reason for the fevers and increasing white count, a drain was placed in the fluid collection. It was old blood; no white cells, no bacteria.

For reasons I do not know the drain was left in. About five days later the fluid from the drain turned purulent. This time the Gram stain showed white cells, mixed bacteria, and yeast, and I was called. I concluded on the basis of the Gram stain that there must be a connection between the hematoma and the bowel. Mixed bacteria and yeast could only get there by way of a perforation.

However, final cultures grew skin flora and two kinds of *Candida*: *albicans* and a *tropicalis*. The heck. Upon further reflection, I decided that this must've been a multilocuated infected hematoma, and one of the loculations eventually eroded into the drain as the clot liquefied. Once the infected clot drained into the pigtail, the fevers and leukocytosis resolved. Let's treat the yeast, I said. And the patient improved.

Fast forward a week. Because of concerns about undrained loculations of pus in the hematoma, a repeat CAT scan was done. I know they always say that they are performed, but that makes it seem like the CAT scan is a musical instrument. Tonight on the center stage we perform a CAT scan.

This time the patient received oral contrast. And what do you know? There was a fistula between the stomach and the hematoma. At some point he had developed a gastric perforation. So I was right the first time: there was a connection between the hematoma and the bowel.

I should've known better and stuck to my guns. Why? There were two *Candida* species in the hematoma. It would seem unlikely that two different *Candida* would get into a hematoma as a consequence of a bloodstream infection.

There is an old literature that you young whippersnappers don't need to know because of H$_2$-blockers and proton pump inhibitors, where gastric ulcers are often colonized with *Candida*. And when the gastric ulcer perforates it spews *Candida* into the peritoneum.

"Gastric mucosa and stomach contents are often an area of fungal colonization, which was detected in 54.2% of the gastric ulcer cases and 10.3% of the chronic gastritis cases. The most frequently isolated fungus species was Candida albicans, although other fungi, previously considered rare or uncommon, were also found. A difference in growth in vitro between the C. albicans, C. tropicalis and C. lusitaniae strains was discovered: C. albicans and C. tropicalis grew from pH 2.0, while C. lusitaniae grew from pH 3.0. This finding suggests differentiation in the properties of these fungi."

I used to see *Candida* peritonitis as complication of gastric ulcer perforation not infrequently back when I was a resident. When I was a second-year resident, cimetidine was released. I am that old. Cimetidine was the most wondrous drug ever invented. I used to get severe dyspepsia on call nights, but one dose of cimetidine around midnight and I was good to go all night long without feeling the need to vomit blood and acid. It was even better than Thorazine for getting me through my residency. Or am I over-sharing? A less important consequence of cimetidine was that gastric perforation from ulcer disease has faded as a problem.

On subsequent upper endoscopy, there was too much blood and debris to see where the fistula between the stomach and the hematoma was. No ulcer was found, but the patient has been on acid suppressing agents for a month now.

One of the rules of infectious diseases is "follow the microbiology." The name of the bug will tell you where it comes from. Not always, but often. *Candida* in the pleural space always means a esophageal-stomach perforation. I had no clinical reason to suspect the gastric perforation, but if I had listened to the microbiology I would've known it was there.

Rationalization

Gastroenterol Hepatol. 2009 Aug-Sep;32(7):499-501. Epub 2009 Jul 4. [Gastric perforation associated with Candida infection]. http://www.ncbi.nlm.nih.gov/pubmed/19577337

Med Sci Monit. 2001 Sep-Oct;7(5):982-8. Fungal colonization of gastric mucosa and its clinical relevance. http://www.ncbi.nlm.nih.gov/pubmed/11535946

POLL RESULTS

The drug that got me through my residency was

- H_2 blockers. 13%
- Coke. The drink. Yeah. That's it. Coca-Cola. 28%
- Valium. 0%
- birth control pills. Them were wild times. 8%
- coffee in the am, beer in the pm. The other way around didn't work. 45%
- Other Answers 8%
  1. PERRY MASON RERUNS
  2. 4 shots (espresso) in the am, at least 2 in the afternoon

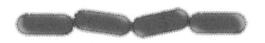

When Is a Knee Infection Like a Lemon?

THE patient has had an artificial knee for about a year and it has worked flawlessly. Until the day of admission when it developed rubor, dolor, calor, and tumor.

Infected prosthetic knee. Not an unusual cause of consultation. Usually a *Staphylococcus* or a *Streptococcus*. This time? Gram negative rod. Hmm. Then it is identified as a *Citrobacter koseri*. Double Hmm. There are virtually no joint infectious with this organism, prosthetic or otherwise.

Citrobacters are a minor constituent of the bowel and a rare cause of human disease, usually urinary tract infections. The patient has a long history of diverticulosis and -itis, so I am presuming for the time being it came from a leaky tic, although abdominal exam is normal.

But what to do? The literature is surprisingly optimistic on gram negative prosthetic joint infections.

"The 2-year survival rate free of treatment failure was 94% (95% CI, 63-99%). Prosthesis retention with surgical debridement, in combination with antibiotic regimens including ciprofloxacin, was effective and should be considered for patients with early Gram-negative prosthetic joint infection."

Although this is not an early infection, it is an acute infection, which is probably a good prognostic sign

*"Treating GN PJI with debridement was associated with a lower 2-year cumulative probability of success than treating GP PJI with debridement (27% vs. 47% of episodes were successfully treated; P=.002); no difference was found when a PJI was treated with 2-stage exchange or resection arthroplasty. **A longer duration of symptoms before treatment with debridement was asso-***

ciated with treatment failure for GN PJI, compared with for GP PJI (median duration of symptoms, 11 vs. 5 days; P=.02)."

I am surprised they cured 1 in 3. Taking a knee out in the elderly is not without significant morbidity, and with no co-morbidities I may have a reasonable shot at salvaging the knee. The good news? Citrobacters complex uranium.

"A Citrobacter sp. accumulates heavy deposits of metal phosphate, derived from an enzymically liberated phosphate ligand. The cells are not subject to saturation constraints and can accumulate several times their own weight of precipitated metal. This high capacity is attributable to biomineralization; uranyl phosphate accumulates as polycrystalline HUO2PO4 at the cell surface."

Accumulate several times their own weight. I can do that with ice cream. Being just across the Pacific from a leaky nuclear reactor, this may come in handy.

BTW: the name evidently has nothing to do with lemons. Citro is intended to reference a citrate-utilizing rod.

Rationalization

Clin Microbiol Infect. 2010 Sep 3. Gram-negative prosthetic joint infection treated with debridement, prosthesis retention and antibiotic regimens including a fluoroquinolone. http://www.ncbi.nlm.nih.gov/pubmed/20825437

Clin Infect Dis. 2009 Oct 1;49(7):1036-43. Gram-negative prosthetic joint infections: risk factors and outcome of treatment. http://www.ncbi.nlm.nih.gov/pubmed/19691430

Uranium bioaccumulation by a Citrobacter sp. as a result of enzymically mediated growth of polycrystalline HUO2PO4 . Science 257 (5071): 782–784. http://www.ncbi.nlm.nih.gov/pubmed/1496397

Flying Pigs

WASN'T that a screensaver?

I had the weirdest thing happen this week. Something I thought I would never see in my entire career.

First some background. I am the only infectious disease doc at three hospitals. 95% of my work is inpatient consultations. I only have three hours a week of clinic. They piggyback my clinic onto the resident clinic and since my billing company charges by the hour, I have no fixed overhead. My time is my own.

Because of that, in 21 years, I have never billed an uninsured patient. I have sent exactly one patient to collections—someone who spent the insurance reimbursement that should have gone to me on a trip to Mexico. I was not very sympathetic. Currently about 1 in 4 to 1 in 5 of my patients has no insurance and usually no other resources as well, so I see them for free. It doesn't bother me, since I don't lose any money by seeing uninsured patients, ID is always fun, and many the best cases have the fewest resources.

I rarely tell patients that I'm not going to charge them. Usually it is only to make sure that they follow up with me that I let them know that they won't be charged for the follow-up. I do not want them to no-show for fear of getting billed. At that point most patients are grateful.

I once had a patient who had been recently fired from his job, and was bankrupt from the hospitalization for his liver abscess. When he was done with therapy he offered me one of his framed photographs of flowers that he had taken. He was a quite talented photographer in his spare time. The picture hangs on the wall in my hallway. That is the only time a patient has tried to reimburse me for my services when they weren't going to be charged.

Despite 21 years of not billing the uninsured, I have never had a patient inquire as to why they did not receive a bill from me. I find that a curiosity. A rough estimate is that I have seen a minimum of 3,000 uninsured hospital consults, probably many more, well over $600,000 in unreimbursed work. I know that the vast majority of people would just as soon avoid a doctor's bill. Considering that I get called in to treat and diagnose the weird and often fatal, with all the asses I have pulled from all those fires over the years, you would think that people would be just a little bit curious about why the doctor who saved their ass never sent a bill.

Until today. Someone actually asked me why I had not submitted a bill for my services. I almost had a heart attack and died. Granted the patient had Medicare, and, probably more importantly, the patient is a retired physician. But still. No one has ever asked before. I suspect that it was due to one of the rare, but expensive times, that I sent my billing sheets through the wash. I hate it when that happens. Work literally down the drain.

Now I'm not expecting a medal of honor or anything. I don't bill, I will freely admit, mostly from selfishness. If I bill them it would cost me money. My billing company is not going to work for free, and I don't want to lose money on the deal. Part of me still thinks that it is my duty to care of any patient that comes my way, since it is not as if the patient has a choice of illness or physician.

As I say, my time is my own to do with as I will. And I always derive a great deal of enjoyment from taking care of infectious diseases. Some people say they like their jobs so much they would do it for nothing; sometimes that's not a metaphor in my job. I once had a whole month with no billable consultations. Such is life.

But you would think that maybe once, just once, someone would ask, "Hey doc, what do I owe you?"

Hey, is that a flying pig?

POLL RESULTS

If the in-patient has no resources
- I do not see them. 5%
- I see them, and bill. 5%
- I see them for free. 18%
- I see them, bill and don't get paid as most of my patients are Medicare. 23%
- I work in a country with universal coverage. Eat your heart out, sucka. 45%
- Other Answers 5%

   1. Hospital pays me no matter what. somebody else worries about reimbursement. :P

....

There Are Some Things (insert gender) Are Not Meant To Know

THE purpose of this book is to make me look like a combination of House (except for the whole opiate addiction thing) and Mycroft Holmes. Almost every case has a final diagnosis. The reason is that there is more to be learned when there is an answer, since a PubMed of the phrase "I don't know" and "infection" yields 5 results, none of which are applicable to any of my cases. Sometimes there is something to be learned even when I do not have a final diagnosis.

The patient is a diet-controlled diabetic who has three days of retro-orbital headache, then unilateral red eye, proptosis, no inward movement of the eye and vision loss. Not good.

A CT/MRI shows pansinusitis (but he has not been symptomatic for sinusitis) and inflammation of the medial extra-ocular muscles.

The patient was put on lots of antibiotics and steroids and I was called. The worry was mucormycosis. As you may not know, rhinocerebral mucormycosis is a complication of diabetic ketoacidosis, but not diabetes, and the patient was barely diabetic.

The patient went to the OR for debridement of the sinuses. The sinus cavities were full of fluid, but there were mostly monocytes there rather than pus, and no organisms seen on the gram stain. Cultures grew scant *P. acnes.*

Nothing to see here.

The headache vanished with the steroids, but the eye function did not improve.

I was reasonably certain that it wasn't infection and was betting on Wegener's granulomatosis, an autoimmune disorder. There are cases of extraocular muscle involvement with Wegener's. But the biopsy did not show the granulomas and, after a long wait, the test for anti-neutrophil cytoplasmic antibodies came back negative. Another great diagnosis that did not pan out.

The headache returned as the steroids were tapered and the eye did not improve, so the MRI was repeated and I went down to talk it over with the neuroradiologist. If you have a good radiology department, and we have great radiologists, don't just read the report. Go down and talk with them. They get lonely in the dark.

Is this, he asked, orbital pseudotumor?

What, I replied, is orbital pseudotumor?

An idiopathic illness that looks just like this on MRI.

We Googled orbital pseudotumor, and I'll be damned (for many reasons besides this) if the clinical fit wasn't perfect.

So the patient went to biopsy of the extraocular muscles and they found...

Nothing. No inflammation, no infection, no abscess, no nothing, and the biopsy showed nothing as well.

Sarcoid and lymphoma are also on the list, and also not present.

So no final diagnosis.

Paranoia rules and I gave a course of antibiotics. What was it? I bet orbital pseudotumor, although not supported by the biopsy. The symptoms responded to the steroids, as if response to steroids ever means a diagnosis. The only disease that doesn't respond to steroids is probably Cushing's.

As the old saying goes, there are some things (insert gender) is not meant to know. This is one of them.

Rationalization

Orbital pseudotumor http://www.ncbi.nlm.nih.gov/pubmedhealth/PMH0002590/

Extraocular muscle involvement in Wegener's granulomatosis. J Clin Neuroophthalmol. 1983 Sep;3(3):163-8. http://www.ncbi.nlm.nih.gov/pubmed/6226714

....

Raise It Up

The swollen leg so shiny and red
How quickly the erythema fades
I start giving clindamycin all the time
Was that the wrong pill to take (Raise it up)
You made a dx and now it seems you have to offer up
But will it ever be enough
(Raise it up raise it up)
It's not enough
(Raise it up raise it up)
Here I am a cellulitic girl
Frozen in the headlights
It seems I've made the final diagnosis
We raise it up this leg
We raise it up
~ Florence And The Machine. Rabbit Heart (Raise It Up). Sort of

HEY. You. Pay attention. I have written about this before, and I expect the entire world to pay attention to my every word, at least as far as infections go.

The patient has chronic, mild lower extremity edema. He is admitted with fevers, rigors, and a cellulitis of the right lower extremity. Arms and legs are "extremities" in medicine. Why we can't say arm and leg, which are actually more specific, and shorter, is beyond me.

After the first day he doesn't get better on cefazolin, then he is changed to vancomycin and sent home on a course of vancomycin, then a variety of oral antibiotics as the leg doesn't improve. Finally he comes to me.

No fevers, no chills, no pain.

The leg is peeling slightly, with a large patch of dark red—the cellulitis that isn't improving. I cure it with my usual technique. I raise the leg higher than the heart and all the redness fades, save for some subcutaneous blood, common with cellulitis.

Cellulitis is never. Ever. Never. Never. Ever. Ever. Ever. Chronic. It is always stasis changes. The corollary to that is that you can't examine cellulitis in the dependent position. The extremity has to be higher than the heart.

Over the years I have cured countless chronic or refractory soft tissue cellulitises, celluliti? cellulitisss? (I can't count very high) lifting the leg up. The rubor, dolor, calor, tumor of cellulitis does not fade with elevation, the rubor, dolor, calor, tumor of cellulitis of stasis does. And do not mistake the subcutaneous blood as infection.

Raise it up.

The Eyes Are the Window Of the Soul. English Proverb

I DO not see many transplant patients. For one, the hospitals I practice in only do kidney transplants. Second, between the prophylactic protocols and the newer anti-rejection meds, patients do not get much in the way of infections. Maybe the occasional cytomegalovirus when they are finally taken off their valgangcyclovir, but that is about it. Not like the cyclosporin and prednisone days, which were an ID employment act.

The patient has been doing well for years with one lung transplant due to sarcoidosis and a kidney transplant from drug toxicity. The patient has a week of fevers, a mostly nonproductive cough, and progressive dyspnea. He is treated with a macrolide and oseltamivir as an outpatient, progresses, comes to the ER and is quickly intubated upon arrival.

Exam: a red eye. No much else. The spouse mentions the patient has had the red eye for several days, with the onset of the respiratory symptoms.

Labs are not that impressive for pathology.

The chest x-ray and CT scan show a progressive alveolitis, mostly in the native lung. Which Is odd, I suppose. I would think the transplanted lung would be the one affected, or at least the process would be bilateral. On the other hand, the native lung is the compromised lung, so more vulnerable?

Everything on the bronchscopy is negative for viruses, fungi, bacteria and acid-fast bacilli. But the eyes have it: An adenoviral enzyme immunoassay (EIA) is positive. The lung is negative. But EIA may not be the best test.

"The sensitivity and specificity of RCA [rapid cartridge assay] in throat swabs were 90% (37/41) and 100% (64/64), respectively, and 76% (16/21) and 100% (132/132) in conjunctival specimens, respectively."

So adenovirus is in the eye and is probably in the lung. Samples of blood and lung have been sent for polymerase chain reaction (PCR) testing; and now what to do?

Back last century, before highly active antiretroviral therapy, AIDS patients used to get cytomegalovirus retinitis. One of the drugs we used for that was cidofovir. I do not think I have given that medication in over a decade. It is also useful against adenovirus in transplant patients, but the big downside it that it is nephrotoxic and once you give it, there is no turning back; it is dosed once a week. How does it work and what is the evidence?

"Clinical studies with immunocompromised patients have so far focused on cidofovir and ribavirin, but prospective randomized controlled trials are missing. Ribavirin is a purine nucleoside analogue with in vitro activity against RNA and DNA viruses. Different mechanisms of action have been proposed, including the inhibition of RNA capping activity, direct inhibition of viral polymerases, and increased mutation in newly synthesized DNA.

It has not been established which one is the possible mechanism of action against adenoviruses. "

But the anecdotes are suggestive, even if we know that the plural of anecdote is anecdotes, not data.

Because we have not grown it, I can't type it, but one last little pearl: adenovirus 14 has been a particular plague of late, and can kill the otherwise healthy people, usually occurring in clusters.

Although this organism is not often associated with red eye, and no one else is infected that I know of. More important than the soul, the eyes can be a window into the infection.

Rationalization

Adenoviruses in Immunocompromised Hosts. http://www.ncbi.nlm. nih.gov/pmc/articles/PMC2570151/

Infection. 2007 Dec;35(6):438-43. Epub 2007 Oct 9. Laboratory approaches to the diagnosis of adenovirus infection depending on clinical manifestations. http://www.ncbi.nlm.nih.gov/pubmed/17926002

Acute Respiratory Disease Associated with Adenovirus Serotype 14 —Four States, 2006-2007 http://www.cdc.gov/mmwr/preview/ mmwrhtml/mm5645a1.htm

POLL RESULTS

The best route to the soul is

* the eyes. 27%
* the mouth. 5%
* femoral, using the Seldinger technique. 15%
* power drill into the vertex of the cranium. 27%
* look at the bottom of the shoe. 22%
* Other Answers
  1. The heart.

Dawg Bite

THE patient's dog was in a fight. If your dog is in a fight, and you see fit to break up said fight, might I suggest you not use your hand. You may get bit, which is what happened to this patient. Right over the first knuckle of the right index finger.

In less than a day it became red, hot and swollen. It was debrided and grew?

Pasteurella. No surprise.

People often think of *Pasteurella* with cat bites, but *Pasteurella* is found in about 20% of dog mouths as well as in rats, pigs, cattle, goats, rabbits and buffalos. I think I would prefer to try and break up a rabbit fight than a buffalo fight. But *Pasteurella* are widespread in animals, and if you get bit it needs to be on the list of worrisome organisms.

One of the clinical pearls with *Pasteurella* is that the infection usually becomes symptomatic within 24 hours of the bite, as in this case.

An enduring myth is that a dog's mouth is cleaner than a human mouth. I have heard this old saw for most of my life. People say it is because dog bites are worse than human bites. That is not true.

For starters, most human bites are one drunk male hitting another drunk male in the mouth, getting a closed fist injury, and then passing out and letting it fester. Animal bites, in part due to rabies fears, are tended to promptly.

And think about it. Dogs do not brush their teeth, they eat their own vomit, and they lick their butts. That's going to lead to a clean mouth? Hardly. The dog's mouth is a bacteria-rich environment.

"Bacteria were isolated from the dental plaques of nine dogs

and a sample of pooled saliva from five other dogs and were then identified by comparative 16S rRNA gene sequencing. Among 339 isolates, 84 different phylotypes belonging to 37 genera were identified. Approximately half of the phylotypes were identified to the species level, and 28% of these were considered members of the indigenous oral microbiota of humans. The 16S rRNA gene sequences of the remaining 44 phylotypes were not represented in GenBank, and most of these phylotypes were tentatively identified as candidate new species. The genera most frequently isolated from saliva were Actinomyces (26%), Streptococcus (18%), and Granulicatella (17%). The genera most frequently isolated from plaque were Porphyromonas (20%), Actinomyces (12%), and Neisseria (10%)."

The world is covered with an unavoidable layer of bacteria, and most of the time this layer is not so much pathogenic as not aesthetically pleasing. But it begs the question, which is worse, a steering wheel or a dog's mouth:

"steering wheels average 41,600 bacteria - compared with only 17,400 for the (toilet)."

It is why I do not let my dog drive the car. Simple rules: lips that touch butt, never touch mine. And when I break up a dogfight, I would use a bat.

Rationalization

Journal of Clinical Microbiology, November 2005, p. 5470-5476, Vol. 43, No. 11. Cultivable Oral Microbiota of Domestic Dogs. http://jcm. asm.org/cgi/content/full/43/11/5470

http://www.autoexpress.co.uk/news/autoexpressnews/202603/steering_wheel_germ_shock.html#ixzz1LKiQNxow"

POLL RESULTS
I worry most about the bacteria
* on my spouse. 12%
* on my dog. 4%

- on the door nob. 19%
- on my patient 27%
- on the computer keyboard 23%
- Other Answers 15%
  1. On that stuff in the refrigerator I just ate.
  2. on the handles of shopping carts
  3. in my blood.
  4. The things are everywhere. Free floating anxiety
  is the way to go.

Otitis Gone Bad

THE patient is young and otherwise healthy. Unfortunately, infections are going through the family. She's a mother of 4, three of the children have had ear problems, and, consequently, so has she.

She has had ear and sinus pain for at least a month, and received a macrolide, a penicillin, a cephalosporin and of course a course of steroids, all without resolution of the symptoms.

A week drug-free leads to the sudden onset of headache, nausea and vomiting, a stiff neck and a trip to the ER, where the diagnosis is 'meningitis complicating mastoiditis and purulent otitis media."

Not surprisingly, the cultures grow *S. pneumoniae*, the most common cause of sinusitis and meningitis in the adult. It is uncommon to see meningitis due to ear and sinus problems.

Resistant *S. pneumoniae* have declined a wee bit due to the vaccine. The Prevnar shot targets the most common strains of *S. pneumoniae* in kids, which were also the strains most likely to be resistant. I was voted that in high school. Most likely to be resistant. And as resistant strains decline in kids, so have infections in adults.

In the 2 years since licensure, widespread PCV vaccination of children has resulted in dramatic declines in the proportion of antibiotic-nonsusceptible isolates in Tennessee. PCV vaccination of children also appears to be a highly effective method for reducing the burden of IPD in adults...

Vector control is so important, but putting out bait traps for children is frowned upon. Of course, no ecological niche goes unfilled, or good deed unpunished, and the serotypes not covered by the vaccine are starting to increase.

The proportion of S. pneumoniae isolates from U.S. pediatric patients covered by PCV7 decreased substantially in the 4 years after vaccine introduction. However, resistance to commonly used antimicrobials, including beta-lactams and macrolides, as well as multidrug-resistant strains increased significantly among respiratory tract isolates of NVS (non vaccine serotypes).

With this patient I bet that given the quantity of antibiotics she had in the last month, the bug would at least have an intermediate susceptibility to penicillin. Nope. Sensitive! Its MIC is 0.03.

Hmm. Wonder why? Antibiotic concentrations should have been sufficient to eradicate the organism. If she had been treated with ciprofloxacin I would have been less surprised. That drug has marginal efficacy against *S. pneumoniae* and I have seen two patients develop *S. pneumoniae* meningitis from sinusitis while on Cipro. Was it a late infection, occurring after cessation of antibiotics? Lack of drainage? Undrained pus is always unlikely to get better. Got me. The host is fine, the drugs were fine, so it must have been the undrained pus under pressure.

Rationalization

Reduction in High Rates of Antibiotic-Nonsusceptible Invasive Pneumococcal Disease in Tennessee after Introduction of the Pneumococcal Conjugate Vaccine
Clin Infect Dis. (2004) 39(5): 641-648 doi:10.1086/422653 http://cid.oxfordjournals.org/content/39/5/641.short\\

Pediatr Infect Dis J. 2007 Feb;26(2):123-8. Increased antimicrobial resistance among nonvaccine serotypes of Streptococcus pneumoniae in the pediatric population after the introduction of 7-valent pneumococcal vaccine in the United States. http://www.ncbi.nlm.nih.gov/pubmed/17259873

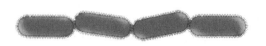

Order Everything, Get Something in Return

THE patient had received his first course of chemotherapy five days ago: the combination therapy CHOP for non-Hodgkin lymphoma. He comes in febrile, neutropenic, and with a new left lower lobe infiltrate. He is quickly intubated and has a bronchoscopy for a diagnosis.

The infiltrate is especially worrisome in a patient with neutropenia, since most of what we see on chest x-ray with pneumonia is due to white cells, and he doesn't have any. So what we are seeing is mostly uncontrolled organisms and vascular leak. Uncontrolled bacterial replication in tissues is rarely of benefit.

As best I can tell, he has no unusual risk factors for infectious diseases.

Is it typical, i.e. pneumococcal, community acquired pneumonia? Common things, I have been informed, are by necessity common.

Is it atypical community acquired pneumonia? Given the patient's age, maybe *Legionella*, which we almost never see here in the great Pacific Northwest?

Is this a neutropenia-related opportunistic pneumonia? It is kind of a roundish, fuzzy- edged infiltrate, but *Aspergillus* et al. pneumonia is unusual with first rounds of chemotherapy and early neutropenia.

Lymphoma related? Doubt this is *Pneumocystis*, but the patient was not on prophylaxis.

Great Pacific Northwest related? *Cryptococcus* does pop up now and then.

So, in this protocol- and order-driven world, how do you classify the patient to invoke the correct algorithm? Trick question. You can't. The patient needs to be treated for all the above while we wait for the results of testing.

In the old days we used to evaluate most patients one step at a time. Get some tests, see the result, get some more tests, rinse, lather, repeat. Now, because the goal is as short length of stay as possible, every patient gets every test on the first day of admission. The "throw everything at the wall and see what sticks" approach. I understand the utility—but, as an example, getting echocardiograms on every IV drug user with a fever before the blood cultures return seems, if nothing else, inelegant. But in this patient, where a prompt diagnosis is critical, ordering everything is a good idea.

And I will be damned (so I have been informed on numerous occasions) if the bronchoscopy and the urinary antigen were positive for *Legionella*.

Legionella is a water bug and I have no good water exposure history from this patient, the *"All Summer in a Day"* weather we have had this year in Portland notwithstanding. Usually *Legionella* is associated with hot, humid, thundershower weather, and that we have not had.

I have to wonder about his shower, and when he awakes, will investigate his water source. Showers are a good source for *Legionella*, aerosolizing the bugs for maximal exposure.

Background: 828 elderly subjects residing in nursing homes were followed up during 4 months to ascertain incidence of symptoms associated with Pontiac fever (PF) in a non-epidemic setting.

Methods: The exposure situation was inhalation of Legionella bacteria while showering. An audit of the hot water system in all institutions allowed ascribing each subject to a water quality area wherefrom one shower was sampled for Legionella assays at the end of the follow-up period. Legionella were detected in water and aerosols using the culture (CFU, colony forming units) and in situ hybridization (FISH) techniques.

Results: Among 32 Pontiac-like episodes, 29 cases complied with the operational definition of PF elaborated for this study. Inci-

dence density was 0.11 case/person–year (95% CI 0.07 to 0.15). Water concentrations greater than 105 Legionella FISH/l and 104 Legionella CFU/l were associated with an increased risk of PF (respectively RR 2.23, p=0.05 and RR 2.39, p=0.11, with significant dose–response patterns: p for trend <0.04). The condition also seems associated with aerosol concentrations above 103 Legionella FISH/l of air. A significantly higher risk of Pontiac-like episodes (RR 6.24, 95% CI 2.12 to 18.38) was seen for elderly subjects receiving corticosteroid therapy.

Conclusion: The water and threshold values identified in this research could be used to inform guidance measures aimed at protecting institutionalized older people from Legionnaires' disease. Immunosuppressive therapy in the same population group can significantly enhance susceptibility to Legionella bacteria.

Legionella has been isolated for hospital showerheads as well, and could be a source for nosocomial infections. *Legionella* are ubiquitous in the aqueous environment, and it remains a mystery why I see so little disease in my practice. It is not for lack of looking. At least we have a diagnosis and can treat while nervously waiting for the white blood cells to return.

In the end? Did fine, had standard Portland water.

Rationalization

Legionella bacteria in shower aerosols increase the risk of Pontiac fever among older people in retirement homes http://jech.bmj.com/content/62/10/913.abstract

Appl Environ Microbiol. 1985 Nov; 50(5): 1128–1131.PMCID: PMC238711 Aerosols containing Legionella pneumophila generated by shower heads and hot-water faucets. http://www.ncbi.nlm.nih.gov/pmc/articles/PMC238711/

Isolation of Legionella pneumophila from Hospital Shower Heads http://www.annals.org/content/94/2/195.short

All the Summer in a Day. https://www.btboces.org/Downloads/6_All%20Summer%20in%20a%20Day%20by%20Ray%20Bradbury.pdf

More Pox to Come

IT starts with a sore throat. A common enough problem in the young, but not when you are 86. Sore throats for common reasons are less common in the elderly. If you reach 85, you have probably been exposed to all the typical causes and should be immune.

The sore throat rapidly became severe and the patient was unable to swallow dinner. Then fever, chills and a rash.

I hate rashes and most look the same to me, and I lack the polysyllabic Latin vocabulary to name them.

When I got called for the consult the referring doc sent me a picture of the lesions, and for once I though I knew what the rash was.

It was a dewdrop pustule on an erythematous base.

So there was Smallpox, now extinct except for in a few weapons labs in the world. And there was the Great pox, aka syphilis. Says something about syphilis back in the day that it was considered worse than Smallpox. *Treponema pallidum* was quite a disease in the Middle Ages. And then there is the chicken pox.

Word origin?

«The word chickenpox comes from the Old English word «gican» meaning «to itch» or from the Old French word «chiche-pois» for chickpea, a description of the size of the lesion.»

I'll believe the first, but unless chickpeas have grown in size, no way with the second.

The third explanation,

"Samuel Johnson told that since the disease was less dangerous than small pox, it was described as chicken."

makes zero sense to me. One reference said it was because

those with the disease looked like they had been pecked by chickens. That is called making stuff up.

The patient has disseminated zoster, and, it turned out, unsuspected myelodysplastic syndrome. Maybe related, maybe not. There is but one reference of the two diseases together on the PubMeds. Dysphagia with zoster is also rare, but reported, primarily in the immunocompromised.

Time, more than acyclovir, made the patient better. We may be seeing more varicella zoster infections in the future. In the old days everyone would get their antibodies boosted as each generation developed the gican pox and re-exposed their parents and grandparents, friends and family. It took a village to maintain immunity.

Now days a combination of the vaccine and adults not being exposed to their grandchildren is leading an aging population with waning VZV immunity and as a result Zoster rates are increasing, although it is debated that it is increasing because of the vaccine.

"HZ incidence increased for the entire study period and for all age groups, with greater rates of increase 1993-1996 (P < .001). HZ rates were higher for females than males throughout the study period (P < .001) and for all age groups (P < .001). HZ incidence did not vary by state varicella vaccination coverage."

and

"When considered together, the differential changes in rates observed by age group provides preliminary evidence to indicate that HZ incidence is increasing in adults aged >20 years. However, it is not possible to attribute the increasing trends in HZ observed directly to the varicella immunization programme, and continued monitoring and analyses of data for a longer duration, both pre- and post-vaccine introduction, is required."

Still, I wonder. Varicella infections are increasing, and, like most problems, the reasons are probably multifactorial. At least the elderly can get boosted with the vaccine and decrease the odds of zoster.

Rationalization

Disseminated varicella-zoster virus infection following azacitidine in a patient with myelodysplastic syndrome. Zhou G, Houldin AD. Clin J Oncol Nurs. 2009 Jun;13(3):280-4.

Clin Infect Dis. 2011 Feb 1;52(3):332-40. Herpes zoster incidence among insured persons in the United States, 1993-2006: evaluation of impact of varicella vaccination. http://www.ncbi.nlm.nih.gov/pubmed/21217180

Epidemiol Infect. 2011 May;139(5):658-65. Epub 2010 Aug 23. Herpes zoster in Australia: evidence of increase in incidence in adults attributable to varicella immunization? http://www.ncbi.nlm.nih.gov/pubmed/20727248

....

Three Cuts

CHANGE of pace.

Mid-50s male, born and raised in Southeast Asia, admitted with recurrent, severe hemoptysis.

Here are three cuts from the CT:

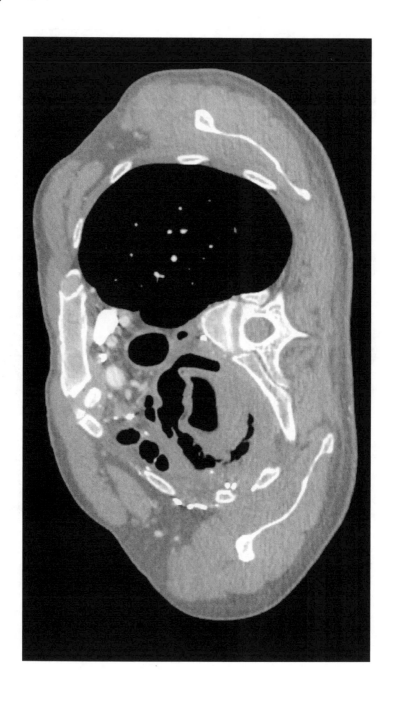

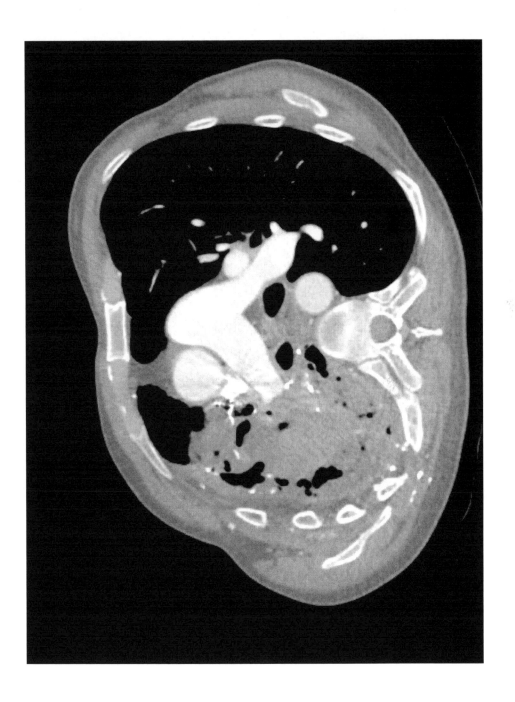

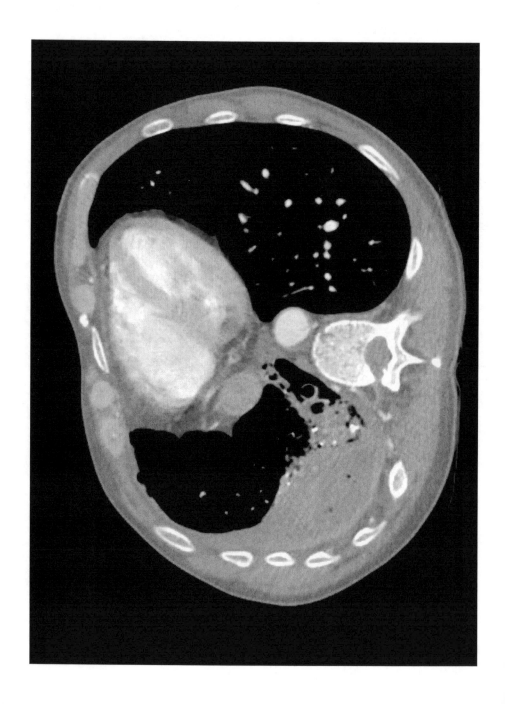

The patient has had TB. He was treated 20 years ago, relapsed or re-infected 10 years ago, and, to judge from the AFB smear, remains a cure.

All the calcium is residua from the old TB.

The upper lobe looks to contain a large mass in an old cavity and the bronchoscopy cultures are growing both *Candida* and *Aspergillus*. While the latter is more common as a cause of a pulmonary fungus ball, I have seen one due to *Candida*.

The consolidative process in the middle cut could be pneumonia, but I don't think so, as it has only grown normal respiratory flora and patient has no fever or leukocytosis. Blood is more likely.

The lowest cut has a pleural-based fluid collection with both calcium and air in it. What it was remained unknown when I left for the weekend.

The bleeding? A Rasmussen's aneurysm, my second in the last year. This is an aneurysm of the pulmonary artery related to a cavitary lung lesion, often but not always tubercular. A pulmonary angiogram showed the aneurysm in a cavity where it was not responding to embolism.

A lot of pathology in a single CT.

Rationalization

Rasmussen's aneurysm — undue importance to an uncommon entity?

http://bjr.birjournals.org/cgi/content/full/82/980/698

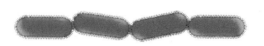

Just So

Iam an Occam kind of guy. I like to tie all the clinical pieces together in one nice package that explains everything. Good thing I am not a physicist, or else I would be forever lost in string theory. My love of a theory of everything is, along with my attraction to an unusual diagnosis, the quirks I have as a diagnostician. I have to be careful that I am not coming up with Just So stories when I come up with what I think is an interesting narrative. We all know docs with quirks, ones who are always finding a diagnosis that seems to be more in their mind than in the pathology of the patient. I just hope my minimal self-awareness prevents me from walking down nonexistent paths.

Like the last month. I saw a patient who had the sudden onset of a huge, painful unilateral inguinal lymph node and felt systemically ill. A day later her upper thigh was red and hot and the patient felt worse. Cephalexin resolved the erythroderma, but not the lymph node. A fine needle aspirate was negative for a diagnosis and the treatment was changed to a macrolide—and then, as rapidly as it came, the node shrank, and was gone by the time the patient made it to my clinic.

Risk factors are minimal: cats (*Bartonella*) and the occasional over-chlorinated hot tub (mycobacteria).

The work-up revealed an elevated white blood cell count of 12,000 cells per microliter and vaginal cultures that grew group A *Streptococcus*. She thought she had a yeast infection, but no yeast were seen on wet mount.

Hmmm.

Any strep throats in the family?

A week before the patient's symptoms, her husband had a tonsillectomy for what sounds like a streptococcal pharyngitis, although it was done at Outside Hospital and cultures were not done.

Group A strep tends to cause outbreaks in families and health care settings. It is one virulent little beast. I bet the husband had it first, then gave it to the wife, although I suppose it could have been the other way around or one of the kids could have been an asymptomatic carrier. But I think her lymphadenitis and his pharyngitis were the same bug.

I have also noted before that leg cellulitis often starts with inguinal pain several hours before the rubor, dolor, calor, tumor of the strep infection becomes evident. I have never seen that documented elsewhere, so we shall call it Crislip's sign unless someone can point to a prior description. This case is an impressive example of the concept.

I tend to think of people like Pig Pen, in a cloud of bacteria, passing germs back and forth—in this case it was all group A *Streptococcus*. I think it all ties together nicely.

Just so.

Rationalization

Clin Infect Dis. 2006 Oct 1;43(7):823-30. Epub 2006 Aug 28. An outbreak of Mycobacterium jacuzzii infection following insertion of breast implants. http://www.ncbi.nlm.nih.gov/pubmed/16941361

J Infect Dis. 1978 Sep;138(3):287-92. Wound infections due to group A streptococcus traced to a vaginal carrier. http://www.ncbi.nlm.nih.gov/pubmed/359723

Clin Infect Dis. 2007 Mar 1;44(5):e43-5. Epub 2007 Jan 22. Recurrent group A streptococcal vulvovaginitis in adult women: family epidemiology. http://www.ncbi.nlm.nih.gov/pubmed/17278047

J Am Acad Dermatol. 1991 Feb;24(2 Pt 2):363-5.

Feeling Negative

U SUALLY coagulase negative Staphylococci can be ignored, or are even mythical. As an example of the later concept, there is *S. saprophyticus*. It is supposed to be the number two cause of cystitis in young women. That is always on the boards, and supported by the literature. But I have never seen a case of *S. saprophyticus* urinary tract infection. Ever. I think it is made up, like the loop of Henle, which has never made a lick of sense to me. I am nothing if not a living example of confirmation bias and the argument from ignorance.

There are times when coagulase negative staphylococci are important. The elderly female I saw this week with a prosthetic knee that had functioned just peachy for a decade—until six weeks ago when she developed increasing rubor, dolor, calor and tumor (I should just call it RDCT). A tap grew coagulase negative staph that was eventually called *S. lugdunensis*. Again.

I may have never seen a *S. saprophyticus*, but the last year I have seen a half dozen cases at last of *S. lugdunensis*. As I have mentioned, this organism is a coagulase negative staphylococcus that clinically acts more virulent than the run-of-the-mill coagulase negative staph. It causes lower leg cellulitis and lives below the waist, preferring the great toe. My patient has severe edema with hyperkeratotic feet/toes that probably were the source for the infection, rather than acquisition at the time of joint replacement. It is sensitive to beta-lactams and has an excellent chance of cure.

The cumulative incidences of freedom from treatment failure (standard deviations) at 2 years were 92% (+/-7%) and 76% (+/-12%) for episodes treated with a parenteral beta-lactam and vancomycin, respectively (P=0.015). S. lugdunensis is increasingly being recognized as a cause of PJIs...Episodes treated with a parenteral beta-lactam antibiotic appear to have a more favorable outcome than those treated with parenteral vancomycin."

Yet another example that, as antibiotics go, vancomycin stinks on ice. There may not be any such thing as a strong, a big gun, or a powerful antibiotic, but there sure are lousy antibiotics. The other patient is not quite as clear cut. Admitted for the umpteenth time for hepatic encephalopathy, he has three sets of blood cultures, all on the same day, all of which grow a coagulase negative staph, not otherwise speciated. No signs of endocarditis, no thrombophlebitis, negative echocardiogram, no reason for the bacteremia. He has been in and out of the hospital enough that it is spiritually, if not practically, a nosocomial infection, and coagulase negative staphylococci account for about 9% of bacteremias in this population. I do not think this organism is mythical either, so the patient is going to get a longer course of antibiotics, probably 28 days.

Most durations of antibiotic treatment are based on multiples of the 7, as we have 7 days in a week, or 10 as we have 10 fingers. I think the Babylonian civilization fell because everyone received IV antibiotics in multiples of 60 and the society went bankrupt. The best way to decrease antibiotic use would be to declare the week to be 6 days long or for every prescriber to lose a hand.

For the record, I treat *S. saprophyticus* UTIs for 11 days with unicorn tears.

Rationalization

Rev Infect Dis. 1984 May-Jun;6(3):328-37. Staphylococcus saprophyticus as a common cause of urinary tract infections. http://www.ncbi.nlm.nih.gov/pubmed/6377440

J Clin Microbiol. 2010 May;48(5):1600-3. Epub 2010 Feb 24. Laboratory and clinical characteristics of Staphylococcus lugdunensis prosthetic joint infections. http://www.ncbi.nlm.nih.gov/pubmed/20181900

Clin Infect Dis. 2002 Jul 1;35(1):1-10. Epub 2002 Jun 4. Nosocomial spontaneous bacterial peritonitis and bacteremia in cirrhotic patients: impact of isolate type on prognosis and characteristics of infection. http://www.ncbi.nlm.nih.gov/pubmed/12060868

POLL RESULTS

I think the following is a myth:

- S. saprophyticus as a cause of UTI. 11%
- the loop of Henle. 6%
- the placebo effect. 0%
- atelectasis as a cause of fevers 25%
- all of alternative medicine. 53%
- Other Answers 6%
  1. All of the above, except the placebo effect
  2. The idea of homeostasis

Atypically Atypical

PNEUMONIA comes in four flavors: typical and atypical. There is the typical atypical, the atypical atypical, the typical typical and the atypical typical. I have learned to say that really fast. There are also unknown unknowns, but usually applies to war.

The patient is a middle-aged (at 54, I think of 60 as the new middle age) patient who has pneumonia. A common illness, but the patient is then ill for the next several weeks, not responding to short courses of a variety of outpatient antibiotics, and is thus admitted to the hospital.

Risks are negligible for any odd infection, and the patient has a bronchoscopy for diagnosis. The sputum gram stain is positive for white cells but no organisms are seen. So it is an atypical pneumonia, and I send off all the typical tests, all of which are negative. So typical.

Then on day 6 the cultures are positive for acid-fast bacilli. Six days to culture positivity defines a rapid grower when it comes to mycobacteria. Mycobacterium is an atypical cause of an atypical pneumonia. Eventually it grows...

Mycobacterium abscessus, sensitive only to clarithromycin.

Not a common nontuberculous mycobacterium, with only a few references as a cause of pneumonia in the PubMeds. It is yet another environmental organism that causes a variety of infec-

tions, including disease in cystic fibrosis patients and the immu-
noincompetent. Oddly, given its name, it most often causes soft
tissue infections.

Treatment is problematic, often being sensitive only to oral
clarithromycin:

*"Cough, sputum production, and fatigue remained stable, im-
proved, or resolved in 80%, 69%, and 59% of patients, respectively. Twenty (29%) of 69 patients remained culture positive,
16 (23%) converted but experienced relapse, 33 (48%) converted
to negative and did not experience relapse, and 17 (16%) died
during the study period. There were significantly more surgical
patients than medical patients whose culture converted and remained negative for at least 1 year (57% vs 28%; P = .022)."*

Amikacin and tigecycline are also used intravenously.

It is the first case of *M. abscessus* I have seen, and I am for-
tunate to have in the community an expert on nontuberculous
mycobacteria I can refer the patient to for a second opinion. A
specialist for the specialist.

Definitely an atypical cause of an atypical pneumonia.

Rationalization

Clin Infect Dis. 2011 Mar;52(5):565-71. Clinical and microbiologic outcomes in patients receiving treatment for Mycobacterium abscessus pulmonary disease. http://www.ncbi.nlm.nih.gov/
pubmed/21292659

Simply Red

As you age you cannot hold back time or infections. Rubor,
dolor, calor, tumor of the buttock and upper thigh. Cellulitis. You can tell work is slow when I discuss cellulitis. But there
is always something to pontificate about, even in a routine case.
ID docs do so love the sound of their own voice, or, I suppose in
a book, the look of their font. A font of information? Naw. Let
us move on. So they started vancomycin. But the fever and the
redness was not gone after 24 hours, so they added cefepime and

called me.

Rule one. And this is supported by the data. Most cellulitis is still due to Group A streptococci:

"Of the 179 remaining patients, 73% of non culturable cellulitis cases were caused by BHS. Analysis of outcomes to beta-lactam antibiotic treatment revealed that patients diagnosed with BHS had a 97% (71/73) response, while those who did not have BHS had a 91% (21/23) response, with an overall response rate of 95.8% (116/121)."

The rest are probably *S. equisimilis* and *S. lugdunensis*. So if the patient has a diffuse erythroderma, no abscess or trauma, start with a beta-lactam. Like Cefazolin.

Rule 2. No data of which I am aware, but in my experience. And the three most dangerous words in medicine are "in my experience." Once therapy is started, the erythema worsens for a day, stabilizes on day 2, and starts to recede on day three. I bet, again without data, that it is due to the time it takes to achieve steady state antibiotic levels and continuous killing. And I bet, again without data, that as the organisms die, their body parts, as they fall apart, incite an increased inflammatory response. It sounds good to me, and that's my story.

Rule 3. Even less data than number two, which says something as number two has zero. Less than zero. Very Elvis. Add a day to get better for every 50 pounds over upper limit of optimal body weight. It is one of my rule of thumbs (rules of thumb?) and I am sure is a hideous example of confirmation bias, but it seems true when it is and I ignore it when it isn't.

Take 'em or leave 'em

Rationalization

Medicine (Baltimore). 2010 Jul;89(4):217-26. The role of beta-hemolytic streptococci in causing diffuse, nonculturable cellulitis: a prospective investigation. http://www.ncbi.nlm.nih.gov/pubmed/20616661

Post Hoc Doc

I HAVE had MD after my name going on 28 years. I have been a doc longer than most of our residents have been alive. Crap I am old. One of the weird things that happens in us old codgers is how much information processing occurs beneath consciousness. What used to be explicit thought has become implicit, and often I know the diagnosis before I know why I know the diagnosis, sometimes on very little data. I often get it wrong as well, but this book is about my diagnostic triumphs, not my failures. Sometimes I would prefer to be wrong.

I usually have a resident on service with me, and as I pontificate on how I get to a diagnosis, I am aware that it is all sound and fury, an after-the-fact rationalization of a conclusion I came to before I knew the why. It is really spooky.

Early in my practice, but less as I age, I would also come up with a diagnosis hours after seeing the patient. I would be home, reading or falling asleep (It can be the same thing with medical journals) when, out of nowhere, a diagnosis would pop into my brain, like a bubble coming out of a tar pit, sometimes smelling as good.

I still, in difficult cases, methodically go through differential diagnoses and organism classes (could it be viral, rickettsiae, spirochetes etc), but this is less helpful as I age.

Last week I was asked to see an AIDS patient. He had a CD4 count of 50 (normal is > 500), an upper lung infiltrate, and back pain with lesions in three different nonadjacent vertebrae. The consulting team thought it was an opportunistic infection. With that information, before looking at the films, I said he is a smoker and it is lung cancer. And so it was.

Now I know that tumor always goes to bone and spares the

disc space. Always. And infection goes to the disc and then into the two adjacent vertebral bodies. Always. I also know that lung cancer presents earlier and metastatic in AIDS patients.

"Compared with the general population, lung cancer risk among PWA was elevated overall [n = 1489 cases; standardized incidence ratio (SIR), 3.8; 95% confidence interval (CI), 3.6-4.1] and in the 4-27 months after AIDS (n = 393 cases; SIR, 2.9; 95% CI, 2.6-3.2). In the 4-27 months after AIDS, risk was significantly elevated for all demographic subgroups, and was especially high among young PWA (SIRs for ages 15-29 years, 10.4; 30-39 years, 6.3; 40-49 years, 3.7). Lung cancers generally presented at an advanced stage. Risk was not associated with CD4 cell counts at AIDS (Ptrend = 0.36). Under plausible smoking assumptions, observed incidence was significantly higher than predicted among 40-49 and 50-59-year-old men with AIDS (observed/predicted = 5.03 and 1.43, respectively) and 40-49-year-old women with AIDS (observed/predicted = 1.88), but not among older PWA."

But I did not put those two pieces to information together consciously. It impresses the hell out of people when you pull a diagnosis out of your... out of thin air. Yeah. Thin air. But it is odd how it is done.

Neurobiology suggests that we make decisions a fraction of a second before we are aware of it. I also can make diagnosis before I am aware of it and before I known why. Makes me really skeptical of free will, and makes me think that the person in charge only thinks he is in control of the brain and its functions. Don't tell my kids I said that. They might use it as an excuse: Dad, it wasn't me, it was my brain. You can't give teenagers an inch.

Rationalization

Elevated risk of lung cancer among people with AIDS. Chaturvedi AK, Pfeiffer RM, Chang L, Goedert JJ, Biggar RJ, Engels EA. AIDS. 2007 Jan 11;21(2):207-13. http://www.ncbi.nlm.nih.gov/pubmed/17197812

Lancet. 2007 Jul 7;370(9581):59-67. Incidence of cancers in peo-

ple with HIV/AIDS compared with immunosuppressed transplant recipients: a meta-analysis. http://www.ncbi.nlm.nih.gov/
pubmed/17617273

POLL RESULTS

I get the right diagnosis with

* medical intuition. 36%
* female intuition. I am female. 18%
* female intuition. I am male and there is no male intuition. 18%
* google searches. 9%
* consulting a specialist, who then does a google search for me. 18%

Unnoticed for a Lifetime

THE patient is in his mid-30s and is admitted to the hospital with pneumococcal pneumonia. It is a reasonably severe
pneumonia, involving three lobes and bacteremia.

It is distinctly unusual for middle-aged men with no risk factors to get bacteremic pneumococcal pneumonia. The easy answer,
HIV, was checked and it was negative. The history was interesting. In the last decade he'd had three other cases of pneumonia,
etiology unknown. These pneumonias were diagnosed outside of
Oregon. He has had two episodes of cellulitis. And further history, obtained later with direct questioning, revealed he'd had multiple ear infections as a child requiring three different placements
of typanoplasty tubes.

Otherwise his past medical history was negative except for recurrent giardiasis. The plot couldn't thicken any more if we added
cornstarch. ID exposure history and risk factors for any infectious
diseases were negative. Family history was also negative.

Now I am many things, but I am not a connoisseur of the
physical exam. The physical can be helpful on occasion, although
I prefer the history and the cultures as the most reliable way of
making a diagnosis. Our Chief of Medicine is quite the physical

exam maven, and he saw the patient as part of Chief of Service rounds. He noticed that the patient had white lines across his fingernails. I would not have noticed them if they had bit me on the butt, although I can recognize some pathology that shows up in the nail beds.

These white lines were Muehrcke's lines. Have you heard of them? Could you even spell it? Or pronounce it? The answer for me was no to all of the above. In case you're interested, Muehrcke's lines are

"paired, white, transverse lines that signify an abnormality in the vascular bed of the nail. Muehrcke first described paired, narrow, white, transverse fingernail lines in a series of 65 patients with severe, chronic hypoalbuminemia" and occur with a variety of chronic illnesses.

and were first described in 1956, the year before I was born. There are new discoveries to be made, and I remain hopeful that even in this eponym-antagonistic world, I may yet get something named after me. Crislip's syndrome: the obsessive urge to be eponym-ed.

The patient, figuratively, smells like an immunodeficiency. But which one? His history suggests that he has a problem with encapsulated organisms. In adults that is usually combined variable immunodeficiency. AIDS is always a possibility, but that has been ruled out. It could be an immotile cilia syndrome, and the patient has no children, but he does not have situs inversus. However, situs inversus only occurs in half of patients with immotile cilia syndromes, because whether or not the body twists left or right is random or, perhaps, due to Chubby Checker. He could also have an aberration in mannose binding lectin.

So they send off quantitative immunoglobulin tests. Everything is essentially zero. No IgG, no IgM, no IgA. The patient has X-linked Bruton's agammaglobulinemia. He has gone almost 40 years without the diagnosis. That is pretty spectacular. In Bruton's, the B cells fail to mature, leading to failure to produce antibodies and resulting susceptibility to infection. It was the first known immune deficiency.

There are a smattering of reported cases of patients who were not diagnosed until their adultery? adultification? adulthood. The disease almost always presents in childhood with recurrent infections, but there is one patient reported who made it all the way to age 64 before the diagnosis was made.

Our patient also had absence of CD19+ cells, which confirmed the diagnosis. As the patient has no insurance, we have not yet sent off for the genetic testing of his Bruton's tyrosine kinase enzyme to determine the mutation, since that is expensive.

It is probably variability in the defective gene that allows some patients to present later in life. I'm sure part of the problem with this patient is a lack of insurance, which often leads to delays in diagnosis and treatment. In this case they would have looked for combined variable immunodeficiency and, like us, found Bruton's by chance. But chance does favor the prepared mind. Louie knew what he was talking about.

Rationalization

Muehrcke Lines of the Fingernails http://emedicine.medscape.com/article/1106423-overview

Br Med J. 1956 Jun 9;1(4979):1327-8. The finger-nails in chronic hypoalbuminaemia; a new physical sign. http://www.ncbi.nlm.nih.gov/pmc/articles/PMC1980060/?tool=pubmed

Clin Mol Allergy. 2008 Jun 2;6:5. X-linked agammaglobulinemia diagnosed late in life: case report and review of the literature. http://www.ncbi.nlm.nih.gov/pubmed/18518992

Simple Disease, Complicated Infection

Even uncommon diseases can present commonly. The patient is 18 years old, is from Ethiopia, has been in the United States for five months. Now he has fevers to 104, shaking chills, and after three days of suffering presents to the emergency room somewhat delirious and hypotensive.

You know what the diagnosis is going to be. Malaria. Indeed, the peripheral smears showed malaria. The patient was admitted to the intensive care unit with a worry this was severe malaria, and started on appropriate therapy.

However, this was not severe malaria. The patient was just dehydrated, not unlike instant mashed potatoes, and improved rapidly with fluids, unlike instant mashed potatoes which always have an odd metallic taste. Subsequently it was found that only 2 to 3% of his red cells were parasitized. Patients with severe malaria have greater than 10% of their red cells involved and multisystem involvement which this patient did not have. A little thrombocytopenia, a mild anemia. But which malaria was it? There are at least six malarias that infect humans.

The patient has been five months in the United States, so you know it's not falciparum. Falciparum usually does not occur more than six weeks after leaving an endemic area. You know it's either ovale or vivax, although most West Africans lack the Duffy antigen that is required for parasitism by *Plasmodium vivax*. But the patient is from East Africa, Ethiopia, where being Duffy positive is common.

"We investigated an hypothesis relating the Duffy-negative blood type with insusceptibility to vivax malaria—and previously associated only with people of West African ancestry—in three population samples of eastern African stock. The samples included Ni-

lotic and Hamitic-Semitic residents of a malarious locale in Ethiopia and Hamito-Semites in Addis Ababa where malaria is not endemic. Fresh red blood cells from 191 subjects were tested with Duffy antisera, anti-Fya and anti-Fyb. Duffy-positive rates in the malarious community were 8% for the Nilotes and 70% for the Hamito-Semites; the Hamito-Semites in Addis Ababa were 98% Duffy-positive. The relative prevalences of Plasmodium vivax in the two study groups at risk to malaria were 2.4% for the Nilotes and 27.3% for the Hamito-Semites, producing a ratio similar to the ratio of Duffy-positive in the two samples. We interpret the data as supportive of the Duffy-vivax hypothesis with reference to a part of eastern Africa, and we suggest that the Duffy-negative genotype may represent the original, rather than the mutant, condition in tropial Africa."

So it has to be *Plasmodium vivax*. And indeed it was. All the patient required were chloroquine and primiquine, and he got all better.

Straightforward, huh?

What I think is more interesting about malaria is the impact it is had on the human genome. For example, when one prescribes primaquine, you should check for glucose-6-phosphate dehydrogenase (G6PD) deficiency, as primaquine can induce a hemolytic anemia in G6PD-deficient patients. But why? Why do people have G6PD deficiency? To protect against malaria:

"Glucose-6-phosphate dehydrogenase (G6PD) is a cytoplasmic enzyme that is essential for a cell's capacity to withstand oxidant stress. G6PD deficiency is the commonest enzymopathy of humans, affecting over 400 million persons worldwide. The geographical correlation of its distribution with the historical endemicity of malaria suggests that 66PD deficiency has risen in frequency through natural selection by malaria. This is supported by data from in vitro studies that demonstrate impaired growth of P. falciparum parasites in G6PD-deficient erythrocytes."

So one would think because the patient has malaria he probably is not G6PD deficient. The rates of G6PD in East Africans is around 15 -25%, although I cannot find data for specific populations in Ethiopia. Still, we sent off the test. What are you going to do, the patient needs the primaquine.

And what evolution giveth, evolution taketh away. It turns out that patients who have a lack of the Duffy antigen coat antigen with neutropenia are more likely to get HIV. Damned if you do and damned if you don't.

"The risk of acquiring HIV infection was ~3-fold greater in those with the trait of Duffy-null-associated low neutrophil counts, compared with all other study participants."

I would bet that there has been no infection that has had more impact on human evolution and mortality than malaria. I once heard on NOVA, and it was said by a Nobel prize-winning physicist so you have to take it with a grain of salt substitute, that half of everyone who is ever died has died of malaria. Personally I believe it.

And, in case you didn't know, there are at least two subspecies of *P. ovale*: *Plasmodium ovale curtisi* and *Plasmodium ovale wallikeri*. These two species can only be distinguished by genetic means, cannot mate, and diverged around 1.0 and 3.5 million years ago.

As a disease syndrome, malaria is usually kind of dull for the doctor, but not for the patient. As a window into human history and biology, it is endlessly interesting.

Rationalization

A Malaria Fingerprint in the Human Genome? http://www.nejm.org/doi/full/10.1056/NEJMe0801414 J Mol Med. 1998 Jul;76(8):581-8.
Glucose-6-phosphate dehydrogenase deficiency and malaria.
http://www.ncbi.nlm.nih.gov/pubmed/9694435?dopt=Abstract

Clin Infect Dis. 2011 May;52(10):1248-56. Duffy-Null-Associated Low Neutrophil Counts Influence HIV-1 Susceptibility in High-Risk South African Black Women. http://www.ncbi.nlm.nih.gov/pubmed/21507922

J Infect Dis. 2010 May 15;201(10):1544-50. Two nonrecombining sympatric forms of the human malaria parasite Plasmodium ovale occur globally. http://www.ncbi.nlm.nih.gov/pubmed/20380562

....

Getting Close To the EMR

Just wait until you are 54. Everything slowly degrades. Laugh, but unless you live big and die young, you too will find 10- and 12-point fonts misery.

You would think that an electronic medical record would be able to increase the font size, given American with Disabilities Act and all, but no one can tell me how to do it on the screens the hospital has. So it's squint city.

All the hospitals in my system are in the process of going completely electronic, so I am on the learning curve, and while I consider myself reasonably computer savvy, as you get older the curve is long and slow.

The patient comes in with a fever. She had been in the hospital a week earlier with a fever which I could not figure out, and then she went home. At the time she had a peripherally inserted central catheter or PICC line due to minimal venous access.

Now the PICC is out, and the temperature is 103, and both her blood cultures are positive for *Candida albicans.* Hmm.Her physical exam and review of systems are not revealing, but having had a PICC makes one worry about right-sided endocarditis. Nosocomial endocarditis is a known complication of lines, and weird bugs like *Candida* are reported. But the transesophaeal echocardiogram is negative. But.

There is clot in the venous system of the upper arm, stopping just short of the subclavian.

So I suppose this is superficial-ish septic thrombophlebitis due to yeast, but there is no rubor, dolor, calor or tumor. No other reason for the candidemia rears its head, and I am stuck with the diagnosis. Made all the more odd as the patient is on warfarin for a postpartum deep vein thrombosis a year ago. Repeat cultures are negative and clinically she is stable as a Dwayne Johnson. Sure not acting like infected clot.

When does superficial become deep? I figure when it reaches the subclavian. Most of the *Candida* infections are deep thrombophlebitis, and whenever I see a sustained bacteremia, I think endovascular infection, which could be the heart, could be a line, could be an infected aneurysm, and could be a septic thrombophlebitis.

For now a long course of fluconazole. But I not yet feel 100% sure I have the right diagnosis, perhaps with good reason.

"Although candidemia and catheter-related thrombosis are frequent, candida thrombophlebitis of the central veins is rarely reported... Despite catheter removal and therapy with amphotericin B, recurrent candidemia and signs of infection persisted, and a complete resection of the involved vein had to be performed. Only 16 well-documented cases of candidal thrombophlebitis of the central veins in adults have been reported over the past 20 years."

Rationalization

Intern Med J. 2004 May;34(5):234-8. High rate of complications associated with peripherally inserted central venous catheters in patients with solid tumors.

Chest. 2005 Aug;128(2):489-95. Risk of catheter-related bloodstream infection with peripherally inserted central venous catheters used in hospitalized patients.

Clin Infect Dis. 1998 Feb;26(2):393-7. Management of candidal thrombophlebitis of the central veins: case report and review.

POLL RESULTS

My favorite part of the Electronic Medical Record is
- tiny fonts. 2%
- chart bloat from endless cut and paste. 10%
- watching the hourglass, the new symbol of infinity. 10%
- realizing the impossible to read handwriting is now revealing typewritten ignorance. 45%

- knowing that to err is human, to really screw up takes a computer. 31%

Odd Bug In an Odd Place

BACTEREMIA is the norm for people. Bacteria leak into the bloodstream in small numbers all the time when you brush your teeth, or floss, or squeeze that large, juicy boil. Most of the time the bacteria have no place to go and the white cells gobble them up. Most of the time.

On occasion the germs manage to evade the leukocytes, find a place to settle down and start multiplying, and disease results. And a good thing, too. If it wasn't for the occasional piece of bad luck, I wouldn't have much to do at work.

The patient has had a bad back for most of his life. Every once and a while it flares, he rests, and he gets better. But not this time. The pain persists and progresses.

Otherwise the patient is the picture of good health, up to date on all his screening, and, outside of daily dental hygiene, no risks whatsoever for an infection.

Because the pain is refractory, an MRI is done and it shows discitis and perivertebral inflammation.

I see a case like this once or twice a year. Someone with a bad back—and the infection always goes to the region of prior trauma—who presents with a discitis out of the blue. The presumption is that the hyperemia and/or clot in the area of the trauma is fertile soil for the organism.

Zenga needs to start an online game: Bacteriaville. You have to start an infection and keep it growing despite antibiotics and the immune system and the end game is to kill the patient. Brilliant idea. I officially copyright it here. My fortune is assured. I digress.

Usually the infection is either a viridans Streptococcus or the ever-virulent *S. aureus*. So we sent the patient for a biopsy and we get...

Peptostreptococcus. The heck. The lab cannot speciate it further, so I do not have a last name for the bug.

Peptostreptococcus is an anaerobic streptococcus and there are

231

a variety of species found around the body. It usually is part of mixed infections, but on occasion you will find it in what should be a sterile site causing a monomicrobial infection.

Anaerobes are not a common cause of discitis, at least as reported in the literature:

"Median age at presentation was 65 years, with a male-to-female ratio of 2:1. The most common presenting symptoms were back pain, fever, and neurologic deficits. The lumbar spine was most frequently involved (43%); an equal number of cases involved contiguous extension or hematogenous spread. Causative anaerobes were recovered from disk space or vertebrae (13), blood (4), and/or soft tissue abscess and included Bacteroides species (12), Propionibacterium acnes (7), Peptococcus species (4), Peptostreptococcus species and Clostridium species (3 each), Corynebacterium diphtheroides and Fusobacterium species (2 each), and unspecified anaerobes (3)."

There is a smattering a cases. Every organism has a smattering. I had a young healthy patient with a spontaneous *Bacteroides* discitis a few years back. We looked for a reason, and no source found, so probably from a brisk toothbrushing. It is why I never brush my teeth.

And it is so weird to be able to give penicillin or ampicillin to treat an infection. So last century.

Rationalization

South Med J. 2005 Feb;98(2):144-8. Anaerobic spondylodiscitis: case series and systematic review. http://www.ncbi.nlm.nih.gov/pubmed/15759942

Don't Pass On the Gas

B EEN almost a week since I wrote up a case. My youngest graduated middle school and my eldest graduated high school. My kids are one of the few things that can get between me and pontificating about infectious diseases.

The patient is visiting Oregon from overseas. She has known endometrial cancer and presents to the ER with fevers, slight disorientation, and new onset of pelvic pain. Her white blood cell count is greatly elevated, 24,000 cells per microliter, with a left shift indicating rapid production of immature cells. They CT scan her in the ER, er, they CT her pelvis, and there is gas in the uterus. Lots of gas.

She is admitted to the hospital, and I am called about 10 am and asked, what is the best antibiotic?

Is she anemic? Nope. Hypotensive? Nope. Toxic? Kind of. How sick is she? Not very. Lucky. She is probably going to crump real soon.

Surgery is the best antibiotic. It is 10 am, might I suggest a total hysterectomy by noon? The most you can expect from antibiotics is to slightly slow down what will be a progressively fulminant clinical decline. And so they did. I always think of work as a controlled environment where people pay attention to what I might say. So different from a home with teenaged boys.

The pathology demonstrated plump gram positive rods and it grew *Clostridium perfringens*. Uterine gas gangrene.

Uterine gas gangrene was a not-uncommon cause of death after home abortions, but is rarely seen in the modern US.

I think the reason the patient did not have a fulminant death was that the infections was initially confined to the tumor and had not quite reached the "real" her, although given the 6 other case reports, that may not be so certain.

Infections and sepsis both result in the production of tumor necrosis factor, which isn't called tumor necrosis factor for nothing. Will the infection help her tumor? Doubt it. But it reminds me of one of the few instances where Koch's postulates were fulfilled, that a direct infection of bacteria can cause sepsis.

I cannot find the reference, but as I remember it, a patient—a microbiologist with lymphoma—infected himself with intravenous *Salmonella* to generate tumor necrosis factor to kill off his tumor. He became septic and almost died. While it did not have any effect on the tumor in this patient, there is a curious literature of using endotoxin and *Salmonella* to kill off tumors, with variable effect. I'd stick with CHOP.

And some serendipitous word origin, thanks to the Wikipedia

"The etymology of gangrene derives from the Latin word "gangraena" and from the Greek gangraina, which means "putrefaction of tissues." It has no etymological connection with the word green, despite the affected areas turning black and/or green and/ or yellowish brown. It is coincidence that, in Lowland Scots the words "gang green" (going green) can be said to be an eggcorn for gangrene, as it describes the symptoms of the affliction."

And now I know what an "eggcorn" is. I enjoy language almost as much as ID.

Rationalization

Am J Obstet Gynecol. 1987 May;156(5):1205-7. Spontaneous clostridia gas gangrene of uterus associated with endometrial malignancy. http://www.ncbi.nlm.nih.gov/pubmed/3578439

Antitumor effects in mice of the intravenous injection of attenuated Salmonella typhimurium. Rosenberg SA, Spiess PJ, Kleiner DE. http://www.ncbi.nlm.nih.gov/pubmed/12000863

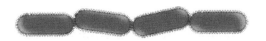

....

Old Unreliable

THE physical exam is untrustworthy. It is fun to discover an odd finding on exam or make a diagnosis based on the fingernails or the color of the sclerae. But negative findings don't amount to a hill of beans.

Two examples this week. A patient becomes septic 3 days after a colon resection. There are bowel sounds and the abdomen is soft. Can't be an abdominal source, right? Peritonitis should cause the abdomen to be as firm as a board. Yet at laparotomy (there was no other reason for the sepsis) there was necrotic bowel and a perforation with colonic contents in the abdomen. So much for the rule that a soft belly on exam excludes peritonitis.

Another consult this week: a middle-aged male with three months of fevers, drenching sweats and a 20 pound weight loss. No risk factors and a totally (at least initially) normal exam and normal screening labs. No nothing. Broadly, fever of unknown origin (FUO) is due to cancer, infection, collagen vascular disease, and other, with infections being the interesting causes. He was sent to an oncologist as initially there was no reason to suspect infection or a collagen vascular disease. Perhaps lymphoma, so the patient gets a bone marrow biopsy.

During this time he also develops severe back pain that is thought to be a bulging disc, but MRI looks more like infection of the disc.

The pathology is negative for malignancy, but the cultures grow *S. sanguis,* a viridans streptococcus. Hmmm.

Patient is admitted and blood cultures grow the same thing. And just after the biopsy he gets a splinter hemorrhage, so the diagnosis is clear. Endocarditis. He has an echocardiogram that shows a calcified bicuspid aortic valve with a vegetation.

So I am called to determine the therapy. I know what the cardiac pathology is, and I will be damned if I can hear any abnormal heart sounds. The patient tells me that the cardiologist can't hear a murmur either, so it is not the fact I gave my hearing to Led Zeppelin in college that makes it hard to hear a murmur.

I usually say no murmur, no endocarditis. Know murmur, know endocarditis. I am so clever. It takes a murmur to cause turbulence to cause platelet/thrombin deposition to result in a place for bacteria to stick.

So we backed into the right diagnosis, but they were initially led down the wrong path because of a lack of a physical finding, a heart murmur, that would have been the hinge point if it had been there.

So I have given up on the physical when the findings do not support the history and the likely differential diagnosis.

I have never made the diagnosis of endocarditis, or any bacterial process for that matter, on the basis on bone marrow cultures except for one case of *Brucella* as a fellow. Bone marrow cultures are supposed to be of help with diagnosing typhoid fever, but I have never had a reason to look.

To evaluate fever of unknown origin, bone marrow cultures are not that helpful:

"Empiric bone marrow cultures showed a low diagnostic yield of 0% to 2% (2 fair-quality articles)."

But to diagnose endocarditis? I had to go back to 1947, where it looked pretty good:

"1. A set of three cultures (arterial, venous, and bone marrow) was taken 109 times (a total of 327 cultures) from eighty-eight patients with subacute bacterial endocarditis. Of the 109 sets of cultures, twenty-four were positive in one or more of the three cultures.

2. The incidence of positive cultures was highest in cultures made from bone marrow inoculated into nutrient broth (twenty-one of the twenty-four patients). The incidence was slightly lower in cultures containing venous blood (nineteen of the twenty-four patients). The incidence was lowest in arterial blood cultures (fifteen of the twenty-four patients).

3. Judging from the mean colony counts in poured plates containing arterial and venous blood, there was no obvious advantage of one method over the other.

4. Bone marrow cultures were positive in four of five patients under penicillin treatment.

5. The data emphasize the usefulness of bone marrow cultures in the diagnosis of subacute bacterial endocarditis. It is to be noted, however, that in some instances bone marrow culture was negative when arterial or venous blood cultures were positive."

There was also a similar case to mine reported in Brazil, but I am unlikely to make another diagnosis of endocarditis on bone marrow again. Or want to try.

Rationalization

Arch Intern Med. 2003 Mar 10;163(5):545-51. A comprehensive evidence-based approach to fever of unknown origin. http://www.ncbi.nlm.nih.gov/pubmed/12622601

American Heart Journal Volume 33, Issue 5, May 1947, Pages 692-695 Comparative study of blood cultures made from artery, vein, and bone marrow in patients with subacute bacterial endocarditis. http://www.sciencedirect.com/science/article/pii/0002870347900860

Brazilian Journal of Infectious Diseases Braz J Infect Dis vol.14 no.4 Salvador July/Aug. 2010 Spondylodiscitis and endocarditis caused by S. vestibularis http://www.scielo.br/scielo.php?script=sci_arttext&pid=S1413-86702010000400012

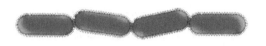

Real, Hopefully Unimportant

THE patient has been down for at least 9 hours before being discovered. Lying on a hard surface, unable to rise, he is discovered by his son and transported to the ER, febrile, with an elevated white blood cell count (15,000 per microliter) and a blood glucose of 500 milligrams per deciliter (normal is around 100).

A workup for a source of infection is negative, and the patient has runs of ventricular tachycardia, so the reason for being down appears to be cardiac arrhythmia. But we interrogate his pacemaker (I imagine Jack Bauer making it confess with some extra pressure), which yields no prior arrhythmias.

Then less than 24 hours after admission, both blood cultures grow coagulase negative staphylococcus and they call me.

No infection symptoms prior to collapsing and repeat blood cultures are negative. We have good residents at Legacy, and I rant every year to the incoming interns that their job is to wake up in the morning and ask themselves, "How can I make Mark Crislip's life better?" The world would be a better place if more people asked themselves that question. And the answer? Repeat blood cultures before starting antibiotics for a gram positive bacteremia. Which they did.

Transesophageal echocardiography (TEE) is negative as well. Now what, since the patient needs a defibrillator.

The bacteremia was probably real, but unimportant. I frequently see patients who are found down and have coagulase negative staphylococci in their blood. I presume the pressure leads to some skin breakdown and in a bad host the bugs leak into the bloodstream. No studies I have ever found support the hypothesis that the bacteremia is both real and unimportant, just in case there is a fellow looking for an idea for a project. Give me credit in the acknowledgements.

Normally I would give a short course of antibiotics. How long? No one knows. 3 to 5 days is usually suggested in normal patients. The closest you can get is a central line infection where the catheter is removed.

"To date, there have been no randomized trials that have evaluated any treatment modality for catheter-related infections due to coagulase-negative staphylococci. Coagulase-negative staphylococcal catheter-related bloodstream infection may resolve with removal of the catheter and no antibiotic therapy, yet many experts believe that such infections should be treated with antibiotics."

I presume the experts run home antibiotic programs. The guidelines say 5 to 7 days once the line is removed, based on zip. I think that is about 4 to 6 days too many in most patients. But how can you go against the all-knowing, all-powerful Infectious Diseases Society of America? No Oz behind that curtain, uh huh.

How do you give a bunny endocarditis? Make it a heroin junky? That's one way. The other is to put a wire across the valve and give the rabbit a bolus of bacteria. With the pacemaker, this patient is the equivalent of the rabbit model of endocarditis. So now how long to treat? With a negative TEE, negative repeat cultures and the knowledge that it is almost impossible to salvage an infected pacer, does it make any sense to give a longer course of therapy? It only delays the inevitable if the pacer is infected.

I am chickening out and somewhat grudgingly suggest 14 days of IV antibiotics, maybe more. But who knows, I bet some readers will have strong opinions, and you know what they say about opinions.

In the end the infection did not return.

Rationalization

Int J Antimicrob Agents. 2009;34 Suppl 4:S47-51. Short-course therapy for bloodstream infections in immunocompetent adults. http://www.ncbi.nlm.nih.gov/pubmed/19931818

Guidelines for the Management of Intravascular Catheter-Related Infections http://cid.oxfordjournals.org/content/32/9/1249.full

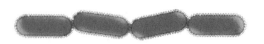

Better Than a Header Through the Windshield

I AM on call. Poor me. If I wanted a convenient job I wouldn't have gone into medicine. The bright side is that in one weekend, covering 7 hospitals, I can see enough infectious pathology for a five chapters.

A year and a half ago, while getting chemotherapy for Hodgkin's lymphoma, the patient was in a car accident and broke her sternum. It was the seat belt that caused the trauma. It was not an open fracture and it was left alone to heal on its own. It didn't. The sternum stayed red and tender, and after a year drained. It was thought, on the basis of biopsy, to be Sweet's syndropme. That's neutrophilic dermatitis, and could have been a complication of her treatment with long-acting granulocyte colony-stimulating factor. I saw a case about a year or 5 ago. But it wasn't and isn't.

Over time the sternum slowly dissolved and it became evident that the diagnosis was osteomyelitis. So off for debridement. Gram stain shows white blood cells but no organisms.

Given the negative gram stain, I was wondering if this was coccidiomycosis or histoplasmosis (the patient has risks) or even an atypical mycobacterium as a consequence of the lymphoma and chemotherapy. If it were staph, the most likely cause, I would expect to see it on the gram stain.

And indeed I was right, and it grew...

E. coli. The heck. Did not see that coming, although I should have suspected a gram negative as they are often not seen against the background pink of gram stained pus. I did not expect it when playing the odds.

Through all her chemo at Outside Hospital, she never had an infection, so I presume she had a wee bit of bowel translocation and subsequent seeding of the sternum. Real bad luck.

Debridement has been accomplished, now she needs a course of antibiotics.

Osteomyelitis is a rare complication of blunt trauma to the chest. Primary sternal osteomyelitis, with no trauma of any kind, has maybe 60 cases in the literature.

"Osteomyelitis, sternal abscesses, and mediastinitis have been previously reported in the literature after blunt trauma or cardiopulmonary resuscitation. Cuschieri identified the presence of haematoma, intravenous drug use, and a source of staphylococcal infection as risk factors for developing a post-traumatic mediastinal abscess. "

In kids there is more literature, again with a predominance of staphylococci, but a smattering of tuberculosis thrown in. There is the usual hodgepodge of odd organisms, but there are no cases due to *E. coli*. I'm first. Go, me.

Rationalization

Emerg Med J. 2006 Sep;23(9):736-7. Case of the month: "bugs are eating my soul"—sternal abscess, osteomyelitis, and mediastinitis complicating a closed sternal fracture.
http://www.ncbi.nlm.nih.gov/pubmed/16921099

West J Med. 1989 Aug;151(2):199-203. Primary sternal osteomyelitis.
http://www.ncbi.nlm.nih.gov/pmc/articles/PMC1026924/?tool=-pubmed

....

Lips That Touch Alpo (TM) Will Never Touch Mine

I HAVE a bad case of RSAD. Reverse Seasonal Affective Disorder. I get bummed when I am inside and the weather outside (where weather belongs) is excellent. The paper yesterday mentioned that this has been the second wettest, cloudiest year on record here in the great Pacific Northwest, but today it is 80, cloudless and I am inside for hours to come. Sigh. I don't need Christmas off. Who needs time in December? But any 80-degree or greater day in Portland warrants closing the hospital

There are diseases that I think I know well, but as is often the case, a patient will be admitted and get it all wrong, and in the process I learn that I do not know half as much as I think I do.

The patient is an elderlylish dialysis patient with diabetes and hypertension who was bit by his dog on the right hand, the side of his arteriovenous fistula. It is loosely sutured in the ER, and no antibiotics are given, being a minor and well cleaned wound.

Several days later the patient is in the ER, febrile, hypotensive and with an altered mental status. He gets the usual work-up, but what is unusual is that the blood lab tech calls the unit: there are gram negative rods on the blood count. And the lumbar puncture shows gram negative rods, with a few white blood cells.

Being able to see bacteria on a peripheral blood smear is a bad thing: to see one per high power field means at least 100,000 bacteria per milliliter. Few organisms lead to this degree of bacteremia. Meningococcus and plague come to mind, although other organisms are reported, including what he grew:

Capnocytophaga canimorsus.

Until this case I had associated overwhelming bacteremia with *Capapnocytophaga canimorsus* with asplenia and the occasional lymphoma/steroid patient. And the cases often have purpura fulminans at presentation, which the patient did not have. The other take home is the relative lack of an inflammatory response in the cerebrospinal fluid with this patient:

"In about half the cases, CSF contained less than 1,000 leukocytes/ microL or lymphocyte percentages 30%."

It appears that the beast has Romulan cloaking technology:

"Macrophages infected with 10 different strains failed to release tumor necrosis factor (TNF)- alpha and interleukin (IL)-1 alpha . Macrophages infected with live and heat-killed (HK) C. canimorsus 5 (Cc5), a strain isolated from a patient with fatal septicemia, did not release IL-6, IL-8, interferon- gamma , macrophage inflammatory protein-1 beta , and nitric oxide (NO). This absence of a proinflammatory response was characterized by the inability

of Toll-like receptor (TLR) 4 to respond to Cc5. Moreover, live but not HK Cc5 blocked the release of TNF- alpha and NO induced by HK Yersinia enterocolitica. In addition, live Cc5 down-regulated the expression of TLR4 and dephosphorylated p38 mitogen-activated protein kinase. These results highlight passive and active mechanisms of immune evasion by C. canimorsus, which may explain its capacity to escape from the host immune system."

Which explains the lack of inflammation in the CSF and the mild, if you can have mild, septic shock.

I wonder, since the bite was on the side of the AV fistula if this was the reason for the widespread bacteremia.

I often see people letting dogs lick them on the face. Besides the consideration of what that dog might have been licking recently, dog's mouths should be avoided. Bad things in there.

Oh, goody. It's clouding up. I should be happy by quitting time.

Rationalization

Ann Biol Clin (Paris). 2007 Jan-Feb;65(1):87-91. Free and intracellular bacteria on peripheral blood smears: an uncommon situation related to an adverse prognosis. http://www.ncbi.nlm.nih.gov/pubmed/17264045

APMIS. 1993 Jul;101(7):572-4. Capnocytophaga canimorsus bacteraemia demonstrated by a positive blood smear. A case report. http://www.ncbi.nlm.nih.gov/pubmed/8398098

Enferm Infecc Microbiol Clin. 2009 Jan;27(1):33-6. Epub 2009 Feb 3. Community-acquired Capnocytophaga canimorsus meningitis in adults: report of one case with a subacute course and deafness, and literature review. http://www.ncbi.nlm.nih.gov/pubmed/19218001

J Infect Dis. 2007 Feb 1;195(3):375-86. Epub 2006 Dec 19. Escape from immune surveillance by Capnocytophaga canimorsus. http://www.ncbi.nlm.nih.gov/pubmed/17205476

Fortuitous Dirts

I DO not spend much time in the outpatient clinic. One hour, three times a week, and most of what I see is follow-up of inpatient infections. Dull. It needs to be done, and needs to be done right, but there are not that many interesting or odd cases in the outpatient clinic. Sometimes I get lucky, which means the patient isn't.

A young woman was enjoying a well deserved rest in Hawaii where, I might add, they have sunshine. I wonder what sunshine is like. Anyway, she was in a hot tub one evening when it started to rain, so she gathered up her children and moved off to the hotel room. Half way there she slipped, fell, and skinned her knee on a wet gravel road.

About a week later it became red, hot and tender and ripened into a bursitis that spontaneously ruptured. She was seen and started on cephalexin after cultures. The antibiotics did little, and a few weeks later it was growing an acid-fast bacillus, maybe *Norcardia*, and Bactrim was started, and over the next two weeks the leg improved almost back to normal.

Subsequently it grew not *Nocardia*, but *Mycobacterium fortuitum*, resistant only to clarithromycin.

I do not think the infection was acquired from the hot tub, mostly as there are few reports of this mycobacterium causing soft tissue infections from hot tubs. The few cases reported are pneumonias. *M. fortuitum* does grow between 30 to 37 degrees, so it could withstand a not-so-clean not-so-hot tub. The patient does not remember if the hot tub was particularly fragrant with chlorine.

The two most commonly reported mycobacteria with hot tubs are *Mycobacterium avium-intracellulare*, where it causes a hypersensitivity pneumonitis and *M. jaccuzii*, which was associated with an outbreak in breast implants that was traced to a plastic surgeon with a hot tub.

The beast is found in water and soil and dirts (I once lost a Scrabble game with a challenge on the word dirts, which I still insist is a plural for dirt, and will try to use it often enough to get it in the Oxford English Dictionary), so the trauma from the fall on the gravel road could have dragged (drug?) in the *Mycobacterium* along with a foreign body to perpetuate the illness.

Short of culturing the hot tub, I will never know for sure. As one review noted, we are surrounded by atypical mycobacteria in all the waters and dirts.

Clinically she was a cure after two weeks of Bactrim, so I opted to continue it for several more months. As a review make clear, there is no standard for type or duration of therapy, but longer is better than shorter and I couldn't justify adding a second agent given her complete clinical response.

Not a diagnostic dilemma, which are the fun cases, but interesting nonetheless.

Rationalization

Environ Health Perspect. 2007 Feb;115(2):262-6. Epub 2006 Nov 6. Hypersensitivity pneumonitis-like granulomatous lung disease with nontuberculous mycobacteria from exposure to hot water aerosols. http://www.ncbi.nlm.nih.gov/pubmed/17384775

Emerg Infect Dis. 2001 Nov-Dec;7(6):1039-42. Nontuberculous mycobacterial disease following hot tub exposure. http://www.ncbi.nlm.nih.gov/pubmed/11747738

Clin Infect Dis. 2006 Oct 1;43(7):823-30. Epub 2006 Aug 28. An outbreak of Mycobacterium jacuzzii infection following insertion of breast implants. http://cid.oxfordjournals.org/content/43/7/823.long

J Appl Microbiol. 2009 Aug;107(2):356-67. Epub 2009 Feb 18. Surrounded by mycobacteria: nontuberculous mycobacteria in the human environment. http://www.ncbi.nlm.nih.gov/pubmed/19228258

POLL RESULTS

When I get in a hot tub I worry about

- mycobacterium. 0%
- herpes. 5%
- Pseudomonas 18%
- Pregnancy. 13%
- what ever was on the skin of the last user. 53%
- Other Answers 13%
  1. Electrocution
  2. How bad I look lighted from below
  3. that fat floats.
  4. getting out

....

EB Jeebies

So much of the time there is a voice whispering in my ear, audible only to me and refractory to the Thorazine (a magazine about Thor?), the time honored trope "There are some things man's not meant to know." A quick Google doesn't find the origin of the phrase, but I associate it with Frankensteen (it's pronounced steen, or so I have been led to understand) but the interwebs do not support that false memory. It is a phrase that will be on the tombstone of my practice. I tell the residents that being an ID doc is learning how to be ignorant with style. And here is yet another example.

The patient had Hodgkin's lymphoma successfully treated 8 years ago and is a cure/in remission. She had standard therapy for the lymphoma and all her body parts remain in place, like the spleen.

For the last year she has had a recurrence of adenopathy. The only symptom is fatigue, but that is long-standing and not appreciably worse. No fevers or sweats or weight loss.

6 months apart she has had two lymph node biopsies that demonstrated the same diagnosis: Epstein-Barr virus lymphadenitis. DNA hybridization showed a modest amount of EBV

DNA in the lymph nodes. What, I am asked, do I make of it? I'm not certain. The serologies demonstrated that anti-EBV antibodies levels were off the wall, so it looks like she can at least make IgG against the virus. Quantitative PCR shows a viral load in the blood of a little less than a thousand. It appears that she just can't quite control the virus, probably as a result of a combination of the lymphoma and prior chemo.

EBV is an odd beast. Besides mononucleosis, it can lead to Burkett's lymphoma and Post Transplant Lymphoproliferative Disease, an odd collection of tumors from a virus. But chronic, low-grade lymphadenitis? I can't find that. There is the acute lymphadenitis with mono, and a few rapidly progressive cases in the immunoincompetant, but I can't find a chronic, mostly subacute presentation on the PubMeds. This is the closest I can get:

To elucidate (Oh yeah, I hate the word elucidate. Long story with mild PTSD at the end.) the latent state and reactivation of Epstein-Barr virus (EBV) in non-neoplastic lymphoid lesions, we investigated 144 non-neoplastic lymphoid lesions by in situ hybridization (ISH) to detect the expression of EBV-encoded small RNAs (EBER)-1 and BCRF-1 and by immunostaining for latent membrane protein (LMP)-1 and ZEBRA. ISH for EBER-1 detected EBER-1-positive cells (EPC) in 31 of the 144 examined lesions (22%). EPC were detected in 4 of 49 cases of nonspecific lymphoid hyperplasia, in 16 of 20 abscess-forming granulomatous lymphadenitis (AFGL), 5 of 25 Kikuchi's disease, and in 3 of 3 infectious mononucleosis. LMP-1 was expressed in 6 of 124 non-neoplastic lymphoid lesions (4.8%). LMP-1-positive cells were observed in 6 of the 31 EBER-1-positive cases (19%). EPC were detected significantly more frequently in LMP-1- and ZEBRA-positive specimens than in the LMP-1- and ZEBRA-negative specimens. BCRF-1 was expressed in 4 of 11 cases examined: 2 of 3 AFGL, 1 of 2 Kikuchi's disease, and in the 1 case of atypical lymphoid hyperplasia. This study suggests that Epstein-Barr virus is prevalent and can be reactivated in the lymph nodes effaced by destructive inflammation, such as AFGL.

Such inflammation may provide a local milieu that is conducive for EBV to enter the lytic cycle."

So is there an underlying problem? No recurrent or new malignancy or other immunodeficiency that we can find. These findings do not appear to be an epiphenomenon of another process, always an issue with herpes viruses as they like to reactivate whenever there is inflammation. For now there is no therapy for EBV, so it is a curiosity, and maybe someday an important curiosity, but as of this writing no answer to the question. There are some things man is not meant to know.

Rationalization

Acta Med Okayama. 1996 Apr;50(2):89-96. Detection of Epstein-Barr virus RNA and related antigens in non-neoplastic lymphoid lesions. http://www.ncbi.nlm.nih.gov/pubmed/8744934

POLL RESULTS

My least favorite word or phrase is

- elucidate. 11%
- actually. 16%
- fer shure. 14%
- dude. 3%
- fer shure dude, actually elucidate. 41%
- Other Answers 16%
  1. Whatever dude, for real? get out my shizzle! Ya feel me cuz u know what i'm sayin'
  2. yu know??
  3. going foward
  4. my bad
  5. It's a mute point

···

Once Or Twice In a Career

THE variety of infectious diseases is part of the fascination of the sub-speciality. This week was I had a first and a second. The second first.

I was doing my daily constitutional, a 3 to 4 mile walk through the neighborhood, when a Beemer pulled up alongside me and the tinted windows rolled down, revealing one of my surgical colleagues. Hey Mark, I have a consult for you, just saw xXx (NotXander Cage) in the ER and admitted them for and incision and drainage of an abscess. Can you see them in the morning? Only my second true curbside consult in my career.

My first second.

The patient had an infected prosthetic knee with MRSA and developed kidney failure from an allergic reaction while on on vancomycin and rifampin. What to do? My order for treating MRSA, considering that all the current drugs are equally crappy, is vancomycin, daptomycin, linezolid, ceftaroline. The real order should probably be ceftaroline, daptomycin, vancomycin, linezolid. All presuming the MIC (mean inhibitory concentration) to vancomycin is 0.5. Once the MIC is 1.0 or more, vancomycin falls to the bottom of both lists. In my secret heart I hope that ceftaroline is tested in real infections—MRSA endocarditis, osteomyelitis, bacteremia and pneumonia—instead of the candy-ass diseases for which it was approved, community acquired pneumonia and soft tissue infections. Well, they are not really candy-ass, but I need a drug that will kill MRSA like nafcillin kills MSSA, and I need the data. Like yesterday.

So I went to daptomycin, 6 mg/kg. Three weeks into her course she is admitted with 3 days of progressive shortness of breath. Chest x-ray/CT shows patchy infiltrates and her white cell count has eosinophilia. Work up is negative for any sort of community acquired pneumonia, and I think this is a case of daptomycin induced eosinophilic pneumonitis. She got a burst of steroids and is improving slowly. We did not do a biopsy, so the diagnosis is presumptive, but close enough for me to write it here.

There is a smattering of cases on PubMeds and the most recent review suggests

"... only five cases of EP associated with daptomycin have been reported thus far, but they should be considered in individuals who receive the drug and develop new pulmonary infiltrates. In the majority of these reports (80%) patients developed severe respiratory failure requiring systemic corticosteroids administration, intubation and assisted ventilation or supplemental oxygen and bimodal intermittent airway pressure support. In fact, in two of these cases persistent complete recovery did not occur and patients became chronically steroid dependent. Unfortunately, we are not able to make any comments regarding the association of the severity of the symptoms and the daptomycin dosage, since the daptomycin dosage regimen was not referred"

Of course steroids are have been tried for every disease and with less than a dozen cases of eosinophilia, who among us are strong enough to resist the Siren's call of prednisone? I have no mast to be tied to, although perhaps the prednisone will stabilize the mast cells and I have gone too far in search of a bad pun and will stop here.

In the end the pneumonitis resolved and the hip was cured.

Rationalization

Eosinophilic pneumonia associated with daptomycin: a case report and a review of the literature. Kalogeropoulos AS, Tsiodras S, Loverdos D, Fanourgiakis P, Skoutelis A.
J Med Case Reports. 2011 Jan 17;5(1):13. http://www.ncbi.nlm.nih.gov/pmc/articles/PMC3033840/?tool=pubmed

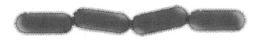

Serendipitous Diagnosis

THESE days you don't automatically get a differential on the complete blood count. Unless the machine says the white blood cell count meets criteria, you do not always get a tech looking at the slide. And that, perhaps, leads to fewer serendipitous diagnoses.

The patient was traveling in central Mexico for several weeks and comes back to the US with fevers, chills, headache and myalgias. Standard work-up is negative in the ER, and he patient is given a slug of ceftriaxone and sent on his way.

The differential, with a slight left shift, was reviewed by the tech the next day and he saw spirochetes. Patient has relapsing, or in this case, not going to get to relapse, fever, *Borrelia* of one sort or another.

"There are two major forms of relapsing fever:

Tick-borne relapsing fever (TBRF) is transmitted by the Orni-thodoros tick and occurs in Africa, Spain, Saudi Arabia, Asia, and certain areas in the western United States and Canada. The bac-teria species associated with TBRF are Borrelia duttoni, Borrelia hermsii, and Borrelia parkerii.

Louse-borne relapsing fever (LBRF) is transmitted by body lice and is most common in Asia, Africa, and Central and South America. The bacteria species associated with LBRF is Borrelia recurrentis."

Relapsing fever, transmitted by either ticks or the louse, has been reported from the plateau regions in central Mexico, al-though the CDC travel site does not mention it and even the Googles gives little information of the epidemiology in Mexico.

Evidently the incidence is low, as there are few mentions in the literature, the two mentions in the PubMeds going back to the 1950s.

Most of the time relapsing fever is diagnosed by the lab tech when they see it on the Wright's stain used to look at a differential. I do not think I have seen a case this century, despite the fact that the organism is endemic in the Black Butte area of Oregon and in woods around Spokane, Washington. It may be due to the decrease in differentials done on the blood counts that has led to the decrease in diagnosis, and since everyone gets ceftiraxone whether they need it or not, the organism is killed off without ever being seen. Kind of sad, really. To live and die and never be noticed.

Twice I have made the diagnosis before the tech based on fevers, chills, headache, and myalgias, that were, well, relapsing.

One case was fun, as after telling me about the three episodes of symptoms I asked the patient, "So, how was your vacation at Black Butte?" The look of stunned amazement on her face was so satisfying as she demanded, "How did you know I was at Black Butte?" I understand the fun that charlatans, er, I mean psychics must have pretending to read the people's minds.

The patient was doing fine when contacted, remembered no bug bite, and will get a course of doxycycline. As I always say, no good deed goes unpunished, and saving money on (mostly) un-needed differentials may have resulted in missing a few cases of relapsing fever.

Rationalization

Relapsing fever Tick-borne relapsing fever, Louse-borne relapsing fever http://www.ncbi.nlm.nih.gov/pubmedhealth/PMH0002326/

Am J Hyg. 1956 Jan;63(1):13-7. A relapsing fever spirochete, Borrelia mazzottii (sp. nov.) from Ornithodoros talaje from Mexico. aje.oxfordjournals.org/content/63/1/13.full.pdf

---

POLL RESULTS

The formally routine diagnostic test I miss most is and can't

justify for medicare billing is the
- PT/PTT 11%
- LDH 6%
- VDRL 17%
- differential 46%
- uric acid 14%

....

I'll Show, You Tell. Part One

I DO not often do unknowns, since it often gets down to "guess the bug"—which can be fun at an ID conference, but maybe not so much for other specialities.

But this one is too cool to not present as an unknown.

Today's patient is a 28-year-old male with beta thalassemia, a form of anemia caused by a genetic defect in hemoglobin. He had a splenectomy years ago and for a short period of time was in an iron overload state from too many transfusions.

He presents with 3 days of fevers and right-sided pleuritic chest pain—a stabbing pain with breathing. No cough and minimal shortness of breath. The pain was most pronounced with he took in a deep breath or lay on his right side, and was in the area of the right diaphragm.

No exposure history or any ID history I am withholding.

His exam was negative except decreased breath sounds in the bases.

His labs were normal except for a microcytic anemia and Howell-Jolly bodies on the differential, proof of no spleen.

Here is his chest x-ray and his CT.

I give you one hint: the findings are chronic and bigger than last CT/chest x-ray two years ago.

I have left out no important historical or physical data. I will give you my tentative diagnosis on the next chapter.

So be an ID doc. Stick your neck out. Gimme a diagnosis.

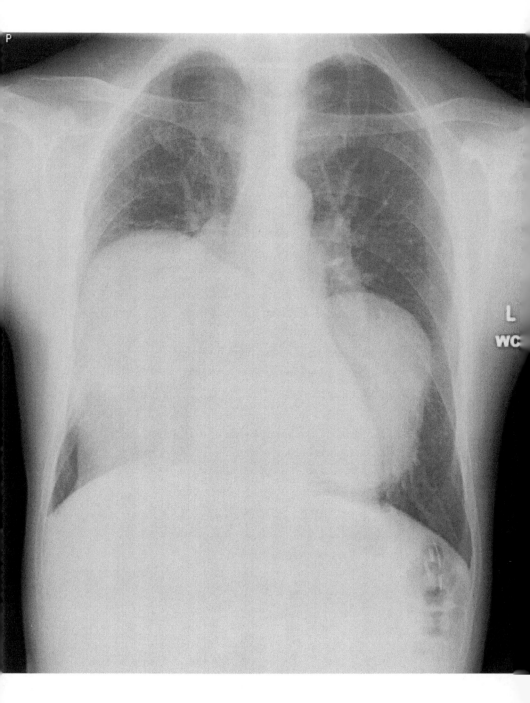

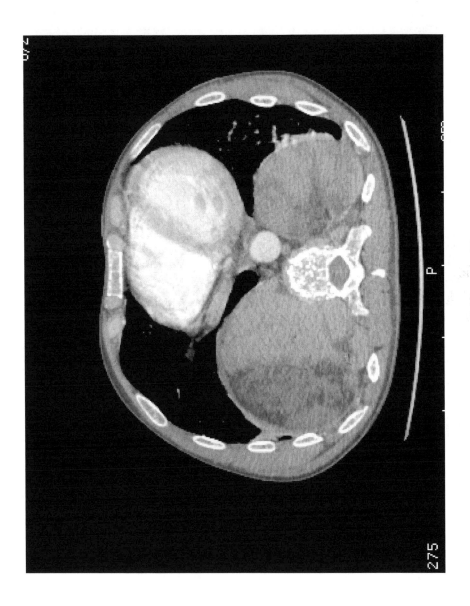

I'll Show, You Tell. Part 2

WHEN I first looked at the chest x-ray, even though I know what the patient had, I thought, "What is the liver doing in the chest? No, wait, that can't be right. Where is the CT?"

It is extramedullary hematopoesis (red cell production outside the bone marrow), so half credit, but why the fevers?

Pleuritic chest pain and fevers have a large differential, but in this case with so many negative studies, my first thought was viral pleurisy. It has many other names, including the wonderful Devil's grip, and also Bornholm disease or epidemic pleurodynia or epidemic myalgia. It is due to Coxsackie B virus, but tends to be a summertime disease, and we do not have summer in the great Pacific Northwest this year. Clouds and rain, yes. Summer has apparently been canceled. (By the way, Bornholm is a Danish Island, not the person who described the disease).

The CT shows that the mass on the right side, where he is symptomatic, is dark on the lateral two-thirds. Could the mass have grown and then infarcted? Dead meat can cause fever, and would explain the pleuritic pain, a syndrome kind of like Dressler's which is an immune reaction to inflammation of the lining of the heart.

So off to radiology to review the CT. The radiologist told me that she could not say whether it was or was not auto-infarction (why I replaced my last car) by CT findings, and could very well be fat. Over time areas of extramedullary hematopoiesis—not unlike the rest of the body as it ages—are replaced by fat. I am going to tell my wife that my problem is too much extramedullary hematopoesis, not too much ice cream and beer.

The prior CT had been three years earlier and the masses had been smaller without the dark changes.

The PubMeds are not helpful for equivalent cases, with one case of auto-infarction, but you know my rule: Never let reality get in the way of a cool diagnosis.

So I call it, and no one can gainsay my diagnosis: extramedullary hematopoiesis with infarction, causing fevers and pleurisy. Close enough.

Rationalization

Br Med J. 1947 July 19; 2(4515): 111. Bornholm Disease http://www. ncbi.nlm.nih.gov/pmc/articles/PMC2055265/?page=1

Postgrad Med J. 1993 Jan;69(807):75-7. Obstructive uropathy due to extramedullary hematopoiesis in beta thalassaemia/haemoglobin E. http://www.ncbi.nlm.nih.gov/pubmed?term=8446561

....

Forgotten But Not Gone

EXCEPT for smallpox, all the old scourges of the past still lurk in the nooks and crannies of the world. I saw a patient today who has probably had active tuberculosis for 8 or 9 months before they stumbled onto the diagnosis. During the time he received two courses of quinolones, and that helped delay the diagnosis. Each time the patient received a course of antibiotics, he transiently improved.

Several reports indicate that response to quinolones fools clinicians into thinking that they are treating community acquired pneumonia successfully and—Oh, wait, why is the patient relapsing?—when they are only partially treating TB. And it might lead to quinolone resistance.

Common things are common, and uncommon things are uncommon. Am I the master of the tautology, or what? But people do not often think of rare infections, and, unless they are ID docs or have a similar DSM diagnosis, they have no need to.

Some uncommon diseases are becoming more common. The patient, a user of various illicit substances and homeless, is admitted with a new seizure. A CT scan of the brain was negative. A lumbar puncture shows 140 polymorphonuclear leukocytes, a protein of 110 and normal glucose. The patient is otherwise post-ictal (in a confused state that follows a seizer) and unable to provide a history. The astute hospitalist sends off an rapid plasma reagin test on the cerebrospinal fluid, which is positive. They also do a peripheral Venereal Disease Research Laboratory (VDRL) test, and when that's positive too, they call me.

Syphilis of the third degree. Lues is not that uncommon if you look for it in the right populations: humans mostly. There are subgroups within the human population who are at increased risk for syphilis, but I remember that people lie about three things: sex, drugs and rock and roll. Well, sex and rock & roll. Does anyone really like the Moody Blues?

Were the seizures from the syphilis, the drugs, both? Some other process? Yes. Who can say?

There are cases of status epilepticus as a presentation of syphilis and one series out of India suggests:

> *"Symptomatic seizures due to neurosyphilis are frequent, may have diverse underlying mechanism(s) and rarely can be the lone manifestation. In view of availability of specific therapy for syphilis, a high index of suspicion is recommended."*

The seizures can be due to gummas, vasculitis, and general syphlitic brain involvement.

He did well with penicillin with no Jarisch-Herxheimer reaction, which is an immune reaction to lysing bacterial products that usually associated with spirochete infections. He also refused an HIV test, stating that he recently was tested and it was negative. And that is always not true. It's sex, drugs, rock & roll, and saying you are HIV negative after refusing a test. Four things.

Rationalization

Int J Tuberc Lung Dis. 2005 Nov;9(11):1215-9. Impact of fluoroquinolones on the diagnosis of pulmonary tuberculosis initially treated as bacterial pneumonia.

Am J Respir Crit Care Med. 2009 Aug 15;180(4):365-70. Epub 2009 May 29. Fluoroquinolone resistance in Mycobacterium tuberculosis: the effect of duration and timing of fluoroquinolone exposure.

Symptomatic seizures in neurosyphilis: an experience from a university hospital in south India. Sinha S, Harish T, Taly AB, Murthy P, Nagarathna S, Chandramuki A.

Seizure. 2008 Dec;17(8):711-6. Epub 2008 Jun 13.

POLL RESULTS (255 in all, the most responses ever to one of my polls. Go figure)

The overrated band with the worst music no one really likes but pretends to is:

- Moody Blues 9%
- Kansas 10%
- Grateful Dead 35%
- Kanye West 28%
- Phish 15%
- Other Answers 3%
  1. Supertramp
  2. U2
  3. Genesis /Phil Collins
  4. Phill Collins

Flight of Fancy

I WANT a reason for a particular infection. Usually there is a risk or an exposure or some explanation for the why of an infection.

The patient is a middle-aged, middle class, straight-laced tax-payer. He has no risk factors for any infectious diseases. Or does he?

One of the upper class neighborhoods in Portland is Lake Oswego. It is a small lake, surrounded by expensive homes, and the patient had been boating/swimming the lake several hours before the onset of first a bad rigor, then a fever, then progressive pain in the shoulder.

One thing leads to another, as often happens with one thing. He has a septic sternal-clavicular (SC) joint. Odd joint to get infected. Usually SC infections occur in IV drug abusers and rheumatoid arthritis patients. He is neither.

He grows Group B streptococcus from the joint, but not the blood. Even odder organism. Group B strep is usually seen in postpartum females (not yet reported in post partum males) and in those with diabetes and cancer, of which he has neither.

I suppose he could have an antibody deficiency, but it seems unlikely given the lack of sino-pulmonary infections that are usually the hallmark of the disease, and his total protein is normal. Immunoglobulin levels are normal.

Here is my flight of fancy: the lake was just recently drained then refilled to fix a sewer pipe. There have been huge sewage spills into the water, and the lake receives a lot of runoff, and it has been a wet year.

Also, where there are people swimming, there is the accidental and not-so-accidental addition of human stool flora into the water. Oregon is (in)famous for having the only waterborne outbreak of *E. coli* OH157, traced to a public lake, Blue Lake, where kids love to swim. In this case I postulate the Group B streptococcus came from the water. Swimming pools can be filled with *E. coli* and *Streptococci*, why not a lake?

Ah, you ask, nice flight of fancy. Any proof? Barely.

The best I can do for evidence is find that there had been a die-off of fish in some lake (not Oswego) due to Group B strep that was blamed on sewage contamination. There is, as best I can determine, no studies on coliforms in Lake Oswego, it being a private lake.

But that's my story and I am sticking to it. And when I go on vacation this year, I am not going in the pool.

Rationalization

Pak J Biol Sci. 2008 Nov 1;11(21):2500-4.
Molecular investigation of Streptococcus agalactiae isolates from environmental samples and fish specimens during a massive fish kill in Kuwait Bay. http://www.ncbi.nlm.nih.gov/pubmed/19205271

Am J Public Health Nations Health. 1928 June; 18(6): 771–776.
Streptococcus as an Indicator of Swimming Pool Pollution http://www.ncbi.nlm.nih.gov/pmc/articles/PMC1580739/?page=1
N Engl J Med. 1994 Sep 1;331(9):579-84. A swimming-associated outbreak of hemorrhagic colitis caused by Escherichia coli O157:H7 and Shigella sonnei.

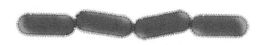

Close Enough to Kill

I T is amazing how the universe keeps serving up interesting cases for me to write about. However, the reason is not because of the bogus Law of Attraction, but because of the number of mesons and anti-mesons at the start of the Big Bang, as is everything.

Today's patient had a prosthetic valve installed 1 year ago, and initially did well. For the last several months has had low-grade fevers and failure to thrive. He went to the ER for evaluation and all the blood cultures were positive for something

It was 4/4 gram positive cocci in clusters. OK, a staph, right? Well, after two days we know it isn't staph. And days go by with no firm identification. Some kind of streptococcus, maybe.

Gram positive cocci are not that well characterized. I think of them as probabilities, like a quantum wave function, and when observed, the wave function collapses and the lab gives it a name. But who really knows what it is.

Finally they said it is *Pediococcus*. Huh. I think I have heard of it. I ask the lab, and they tell me they tried to ID it twice and got a different result each time. Different wave function collapse each time? It has the right biochemicals and is vancomycin resistant. So *Pediococcus* it is.

"The pediococci were first discovered in food products such as beer, cheese, meats, and plants...two reported cases of endocarditis, four patients had sepsis, two patients were reported with peritonitis, and the remaining nine blood cultures were from bacteremic patients."

So not so common. What to do? It is sensitive to penicillin, so I can kill it. I hope. One never knows with a prosthetic valve infection. The TEE did not show any evil like a ring abscess, so maybe the patient will get lucky.

They did. Call it a cure.

Rationalization

Clin Microbiol Rev. 1995 Oct;8(4):479-95. Identification, classification, and clinical relevance of catalase-negative, gram-positive cocci,
excluding the streptococci and enterococci. http://www.ncbi.nlm.nih.
gov/pmc/articles/PMC172872/pdf/080479.pdf

How Low Can You Go?

I HAVE actually been off for a week, at a conference in Las Vegas,
giving talks. You know the Vegas motto: what happens in Vegas stays as a purulent ulcer. Or something like that. Did you miss
me? Really? You are not just saying that to make me feel good are
you? You are? Sigh.

Back to work. The lowest hemoglobin (Hgb) I have ever seen
due to an infectious disease was 3.0 milligrams per deciliter from
Mycoplasma-induced hemolytic anemia. The patient was tired
and very pale, even for an Oregonian or a vampire, but otherwise
asymptomatic. Pretty impressive, since the lower limit of normal
is 12-13. It pays to be 18 years old; they tolerate pathology more
than old geezers.

The patient today is in his mid-thirties and comes in with fevers, shortness of breath, nonproductive cough, malaise and his
Hgb was quite low at 8, making him anemic. We investigated
the cause of the anemia by measuring his lactate dehydrogenase
(LDH) levels, a marker of red cell lysis. His value was 1110 international units per liter, almost six times the upper limit of normal. His reticulocyte count was 5.5%, when about 1% is normal.
Reticulocytes are immature red cells. So his red blood cells were
lysing, and his bone marrow was working overtime to try to com-
pensate. Hemolytic anemia.

More interesting is that he had been in the hospital a week
prior with the diagnosis of "viral" myocarditis, and with troponins
(a measure of heart muscle injury) of 14 ng/mL, very highly elevated. Normal is 0-0.4 ng/mL. His Hgb at the time was also
14 (milligrams per deciliter, in this case), which was normal. The

residents assure me the troponin is abnormal. Back in my day, before such nonsense as troponins, we diagnosed cardiac injury with LDH isoenzymes. Ha. We were real doctors.

The chest x-ray is not that impressive, but his cold agglutinins were high, so ID was involved. Is this *Mycoplasma?*

Could be. It would be one of the classic extrapulmonary manifestations and I suggested everyone read *"The protean manifestations of Mycoplasma pneumoniae infection in adults"* a classic in the world of infectious diseases. Not *To Kill a Mockingbird* classic, but as close as ID gets.

I would like it to be *Mycoplasma,* but there has been a distinct lack of pneumonia on x-ray, although one review says

"Extrapulmonary complications may present before, during, after, or in the absence of pulmonary signs."

Other diseases are reported, most interestingly Coxsackievirus B infection, where the hemolytic anemia occurred several weeks after the myocarditis and in the few reported cases of *Mycoplasma* where the carditis and anemia occurred simultaneously. EBV, CMV and typhoid fever are also on the list with a case report each, but no travel and no compatible clinical syndrome.

So we wait for the *Mycoplasma* tests as his Hgb hits 5.0. Not a record, but I do not want to set one. Hematology, of course, is doing their magic to keep the hemolysis at bay. All medicine that is not antibiotics is more or less magic to me.

The IgM was postive for *Mycoplasma* and he eventually got all better.

Rationalization

Am J Med. 1975 Feb;58(2):229-42. The protean manifestations of Mycoplasma pneumoniae infection in adults. http://www.ncbi.nlm.nih.gov/pubmed/163580

Braz J Infect Dis. 2009 Feb;13(1):77-9. Mycoplasma pneumoniae associated with severe autoimmune hemolytic anemia: case report and literature review. http://www.ncbi.nlm.nih.gov/pubmed/19578637

Infectious Diseases in Clinical Practice November 2010 - Volume

18 - Issue 6 - pp 408-410 Autoimmune Hemolytic Anemia in Acute
Coxsackievirus B Infection http://journals.lww.com/infectious/Ab-
stract/2010/11000/Autoimmune_Hemolytic_Anemia_in_Acute.15.
aspx

POLL RESULTS
In my mind, 'how low can you go?' refers to
- Hgb. 0%
- Diving. 6%
- Vegas after a pint or two of rum. 12%
- Republican politics. 53%
- Democratic politics. 12%
- Other Answers 18%
    1. Not any where near the beer so we could buy you some!
    2. Limbo

....

Imagine

STAPHYLOCOCCUS aureus pays my mortgage.
At least it would if most of my patients had something
other than medicare or no insurance. But in a perfect world, staph
would pay my mortgage, although I suppose for those other than
infectious disease doctors, a perfect world would not have staph
infections.

Right now most of my service consists of *S. aureus* infections:
wound infections, bacteremia, septic joints, endocarditis etc.
Some MRSA, some MSSA.

In my hypothetically perfect world, what to do is simple. Depending on the infection, patients need a reasonably well defined
course of an IV anti-staphylococcal beta-lactam, and then, perhaps, a course of oral antibiotics depending on the infection and
the response.

In a non perfect world I have a lack of payers, IV drug abusers—er, sorry, the term now is injection drug users—and many a
patient who does not want to participate in their treatment plan,
which may include coming into the clinic for their infusions.

What is a mother to do? Once you can't give cefazolin or oxacillin, all other options are inferior.

Once a day ceftriaxone is inferior to the first generation cephalosporins.

"Treatment of MSSA bacteraemia with cefazolin is not significantly different from treatment with cloxacillin, while treatment with other beta-lactams, including second and third generation cephalosporins, might be associated with higher mortality."

All non-beta lactams, vancomycin, daptomycin, linezolid, tigecycline and the ultimate worthless antibiotic, Synercid, are less effective than beta-lactams.

It would be nice to treat the recalcitrant homeless IV drug abusers with oral agents, and both quinolone/rifampin and TMP/Sulfa/ with maybe rifampin look as promising as vancomycin for non-endocarditis, i.e. only modestly crappy.

What the world needs is a once a week IV anti-staphylococcal beta-lactam that kills MSSA and MRSA that costs a dollar a dose. In the meantime I will juggle options with the limitations of funding, heroin, and the occasional sociopathy.

Imagine. John Lennon wasn't even close.

Rationalization

J Antimicrob Chemother. 2010 Aug;65(8):1779-83. Epub 2010 May 27. Co-trimoxazole versus vancomycin for the treatment of methicillin-resistant Staphylococcus aureus bacteraemia: a retrospective cohort study. http://www.ncbi.nlm.nih.gov/pubmed/20507860

Clin Microbiol Infect. 2010 Nov 13. Are all beta-lactams similarly effective in the treatment of methicillin-sensitive Staphylococcus aureus bacteraemia? http://www.ncbi.nlm.nih.gov/pubmed/21073629

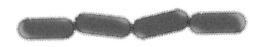

Bad Luck

Patients like to have answers, as do I. Why did they get a particular infection? I can often sort of answer the question, knowing the epidemiology and physiology. But in the end it often comes down to bad luck. Why that bug in that body space at that time and place? Bad luck.

And patients virtually always respond, with a perverse sort of pride, "That's typical—if something bad is going to happen, something unusual, it is going to happen to me." No one has ever said, "That is just so weird, I have always been lucky, and that kind of thing never happens to me." Everyone has bad luck, no one, it seems, has good luck. Except me. My life so far has been one long run of good luck, so I suppose I will never get an unusual infection

The patient had bad luck a couple of years ago: prosthetic valve endocarditis with a *Streptococcus salivarius*. I cured it. Well, the antibiotics did. But I suggested them, so I get at least partial credit.

She was doing fine when she developed a prolonged coughing illness. Sounds like it was pertussis, but she never had a diagnosis. Persistent coughing led to a slowly increasing abdominal mass, a hernia, in an old surgical hernia repair site. Bad luck, it grew to the size of a baseball.

Then it became red, hot, and extremely painful. The diagnosis was an incarcerated hernia with question of strangulated bowel. Not a good diagnosis; more bad luck.

But in the OR no strangulated bowel was found, but an infected seroma. Cultures grew another oral streptococcus, just like the endocarditis all those many years ago. Like the endocarditis, the seroma was probably seeded from the mouth. So it wasn't dead bowel, but an easily treated streptococcal abscess. Good luck or bad luck? Half full or half empty? Optimist or pessimist? Jiff or Skippy?

But that begged the question, just what is a seroma? A song by the Knack?

Da da da da dum da dum da dum da My Seroma. Bit of a stretch?

Seromas are fluid collections after surgery, but why to they form and what to do about them?

I can't find much. Seromas are common after hernia repairs with mesh placement, much like this patient had, and after other surgeries. There does not appear to be a standard approach for their prevention. And while infections and seromas can occur with surgery, a PubMed search for infected seromas yielded nothing. So this would be, I suppose, real bad luck. Or so mundane as to not be worth reporting. Doesn't stop me.

References

Scand J Surg. 2010;99(1):24-7. Seroma formation and method of mesh fixation in laparoscopic ventral hernia repair—highlights of a case series. http://www.ncbi.nlm.nih.gov/pubmed/20501354

....

SOS DD

SAME old staph, different day. It is never the same old staph. This has been a week of *S. aureus*.

First case was a multifocal, necrotizing pneumonia that relapsed after a course of vancomycin. Multiple abscesses with air fluid levels, but the vancomycin MIC went from 1.0 to 2.0 over the last two weeks. As the vancomycin MIC creeps up, the success rate with vancomycin falls. So what to treat the patient with? I opted for ceftaroline and she responded very quickly to the treatment. I sure wish we had some clinical trials with ceftaroline and MRSA so I really knew how good it really is. My sense is it's really good, much better than vancomycin, but then damn near anything would be better than vancomycin. One of the new residents said they were really into using linezolid at their institution, but I have never been enamored with the drug. Too costly and toxic and not that much better than vancomycin.

"Our study does not demonstrate clinical superiority of linezolid vs. glycopeptides for the treatment of nosocomial pneumonia despite a statistical power of 95%. Linezolid shows a significant two-fold increase in the risk of thrombocytopenia and gastrointestinal events. Vancomycin and teicoplanin are not associated with more renal dysfunction than linezolid."

The next was a young IV drug abuser, who came in with MSSA bacteremia and a tricuspid valve vegetation. After two doses of antibiotics she left AMA (against medical advice) for heroin and returned 9 days later very sick. It is not good to let your endocarditis fester for several weeks. The chest x-ray shows multiple septic lung emboli as well. If she stays with the plan this time, maybe we will cure it. Otherwise, death is in her future. I fret about a myocardial abscess, and will probably get a transesophageal echocardiogram if she will let us.

She didn't, leaving AMA again, never to return.

The last was an older person with a new aortic valve 3 three months ago and a pacer system 3 years ago with two days of fevers and chills, who presents to Outside Hospital with MRSA in the blood. Exam is less than impressive for a source of the infection, so it is probably an infection of either the valve or pacer, despite a negative TEE.

"Of the 62 patients with SAB and a CIED, 22 patients (35.5%) had CIED infection. The generator pocket was identified as the source of bacteremia in seven (11%) patients. The majority of CIED infections were device-related infective endocarditis (12 of 22, 55%). Thirty percent of patients presenting with SAB greater than 1 year after device implantation had CIED infection; all but one had CIED-related infective endocarditis. Sixty percent of ICD patients (12 of 20) with SAB had CIED infection, compared with 24% of PPM patients (10 of 42, P = 0.01). On univariate analysis factors associated with CIED-related infective endocarditis included device type [odds ratio (OR) for

ICD 13.3, 95% confidence interval [CI] 2.1, 84.9) and presence of a prosthetic heart valve (OR 6.8 95% CI 1.1, 43.4). CONCLUSIONS: CIED infection is common in patients with SAB. The presence of an ICD and prosthetic heart valve were associated with CIED-related infective endocarditis. Subsequent work should focus on prospectively characterizing the subset of patients with CIED infection who present with SAB as the sole manifestation of their device infection. (PACE 2010; 407-413)."

and

"In this investigation, approximately half of all patients with prosthetic valves who developed S. aureus bacteremia had definite endocarditis."

So he is heading for a long course of antibiotics, although if the pacer system is involved, there is little chance of cure. As an aside, I have long postulated that patients on Coumadin, as was the case in this patient, will be less likely to have vegetations on echocardiography since they can't make clot, and vegetations are largely clot. No one has yet to do the study—so for any budding cardiologists, get to work. Give me credit in the thanks.

BTW: In a self-serving postscript, there are now at least three studies, all done by ID docs, that show improved outcomes in patients with *S. aureus* bacteremia who get ID consults. Don't try it at home, hire a professional.

Rationalization

Crit Care Med. 2010 Sep;38(9):1802-8 Linezolid versus vancomycin or teicoplanin for nosocomial pneumonia: a systematic review and meta-analysis. http://www.ncbi.nlm.nih.gov/pubmed/20639754

Pacing Clin Electrophysiol. 2010 Apr;33(4):407-13. Epub 2009 Sep 30. Cardiovascular implantable electronic device infection in patients with Staphylococcus aureus bacteremia. http://www.ncbi.nlm.nih.gov/pubmed/19793360

Am J Med. 2005 Mar;118(3):225-9. Risk of endocarditis among patients with prosthetic valves and Staphylococcus aureus bacteremia. http://www.ncbi.nlm.nih.gov/pubmed/15745719

The Return of the King

Guess who's back, back again
Crislip's back, tell a friend
Guess who's back, guess who's back,
Guess who's back, guess who's back,
..Now this looks like a job for me
So everybody just follow me
Cuz we need a little controversy
Cuz it feels so empty without me.

VACATIONS are great. The first couple of days back? Not so much. I don't know the patients, decisions and mail have piled up, and mentally, well, it is amazing how quickly the brain stops firing on all cylinders and how long it takes to get running smoothly again. What I need is a WD-40 for the brain. Maybe beer, but that is contraindicated at work.

Endocarditis is a relatively common disease in my practice, and I have had a flurry of cases of late. Is flurry the collective noun for endocarditis? Maybe a vegetation of endocarditis? One was a *Streptococcus mitis* aortic valve endocarditis that may or may not have occurred just after dental work. It had a slightly high MIC to penicillin, 0.1, but he did well clinically.

At follow up he had developed new neck pain that was not mentioned in the hospital. It was on the right—he pointed to where a vampire might start a sip—but he had good range of motion, did not require narcs, and had no point tenderness on the spine. There was also a lovely (for a doc) diastolic blowing murmur. You don't get to hear those all that often. It does not appear to be a discitis or vertebral osteomyelitis, but still. Bacteremia and neck pain makes one nervous.

So off to the MRI and it showed that there were changes consistent with a cervical facet joint arthritis/transverse process osteomyelitis.

Weird. I have seen one other in my career, a *Streptococcus viridans* that occurred after dental work, but her risk had been radiation of her tonsils and acne back in the bad old days when the answer to many processes was "radiate." This patient had no reason for an osteomyelitis in that part of the spine, except for bacteremia from endocarditis. I suppose it could have been an embolic event.

There are a smattering of reports in humans on the PubMeds and facet joint infection can occur after both direct inoculation from epidurals and acupuncture, as well as hematogenously. Lumbar disease seems to predominate:

"Two retrospective reviews of case reports in the literature found that septic arthritis of the facet joint causes 4-20% of pyogenic spinal infections, the average patient age is 55-59 and the overwhelming majority, 86-97%, occur in the lumbar spine. While most cases are thought to occur via hematogenous spread, there are a number of case reports in the literature where septic arthritis of the facet joint resulted from iatrogenic causes including corticosteroid injection3,7and epidural catheterization. These infections can also occur secondary to spread from adjacent infections such as spondylodiscitis, epidural or paraspinal abscess, psoas muscle abscess or other intraabdominal infections."

With that finding I will extend the duration of antibiotics to 6 weeks. It goes to show you the importance of looking for answers rather than treating.

Rationalization

Iowa Orthop J. 2010;30:182-7. Cervical facet joint septic arthritis: a case report. http://www.ncbi.nlm.nih.gov/pubmed/21045995

Acupunct Med. 2004 Sep;22(3):152-5. Unilateral septic arthritis of a lumbar facet joint secondary to acupuncture treatment—a case report. http://www.ncbi.nlm.nih.gov/pubmed/15551942

....

Peripheral IVz: Homines Non Boni Seriose

THERE are numerous events that let me know that I am an out-of-touch old geezer, ready to be set loose on an iceberg, and don't think for a moment I am not glad for a touch of global warming taking that option out of the hands of my children.

House staff keep coming up with new abbreviations, and I do not know where they come from. "PNA" has come out of nowhere in the last few years as a substitution for pneumonia. Is that West Coast deal, or do they use it in the rest of the world? It seems like such an awkward abbreviation. The abbreviations may change, but at least the infections stay the same.

The patient recently has fevers and chills and is ill. So his spouse, as spouses are wont to do, brings him to the ER, and a good thing too. After the usual fever work up (he had no "PNA") all his blood cultures grow MSSA. The source appears to be a recent IV site that went bad. One of the first deaths I saw, back when I was an intern, was a *S. aureus* bacteremia from a peripheral vein that seeded the aortic valve and then blew out the valve. Staph has a nasty propensity of going places like heart valves, although to judge from clinical response, repeat negative blood cultures, and an ECHO, his valves are (probably) spared.

We spend a lot of time and energy trying to prevent central catheter infections, but peripheral IVs have the same potential to be a source of infection. IV teams help, but how often should peripheral IVs be changed? When randomized to scheduled replacement or waiting for a reason to change the peripheral IV, there was no difference in infection or complication rates.

"There is growing evidence to support the extended use of peripheral IVDs with removal only on clinical indication."

Which kind of surprises me, although that is why clinical

studies are necessary. Personal experience is worthless as a guide to therapy. Still, to paraphrase me, the true axis of evil is the Foley, the IV, and poor hand hygiene, at least for now. Unfortunately none are amenable to armed intervention.

While his valves were spared, when his mental status improved he noted that he had more floaters in his vision than before he became ill. Ophthalmology took a look in his eyes and he has bilateral endopthalmitis—only the second time I have seen this from *S. aureus* in 25 years. Bilateral eye involvement is uncommon and often associated with a bad outcome. His is, fortunately, mild, but my other patient lost all vision due to the infection.

Take-homes? Or should it be takes home? IVs should be used sparingly, *S. aureus* loves to cause metastatic complications in odd places so pay attention to new symptoms in patients with bacteremia.

Rationalization

BMC Med. 2010 Sep 10;8:53. Routine resite of peripheral intravenous devices every 3 days did not reduce complications compared with clinically indicated resite: a randomized controlled trial. Rickard CM, McCann D, Munnings J, McGrail MR. http://www.ncbi.nlm. nih.gov/pubmed/20831782

South Med J. 2009 Sep;102(9):952-6. SAME is different: a case report and literature review of Staphylococcus aureus metastatic endophthalmitis. Nixdorff NA, Tang J, Mourad R, Skalweit MJ. http:// www.ncbi.nlm.nih.gov/pubmed/19668027

Acta Ophthalmol Scand. 2004 Jun;82(3 Pt 1):306-10. Bilateral endogenous bacterial endophthalmitis: a report of four cases. http:// www.ncbi.nlm.nih.gov/pubmed/15115453

A First, After All These Years

I HAVE been slogging away in the ID trenches for 25 years and there appears to be almost too numerous to count diseases and processes that I have yet to see. Like this week, a first.

The patient is a young male, returned from Africa from a stint in the Peace Corps. As part of his decommissioning, he has a skin tuberculin test (PPD) placed, It is a whopping positive, and he is referred to me.

No signs of TB, chest x-ray is clear, we discuss the pros and cons of the anti-TB antibiotic isoniazid (INH) and decide in favor of 9 months of INH.

Three months later he presents with fatigue and a day of right upper quadrant tenderness, but the exam is normal. So liver function tests are checked and indeed they are elevated, about 6 times normal.

Hepatitis is a well known complication of INH but in all the years of killing TB, this is my first case.

20% or so of patients will get a 2-3 fold increase in the liver function tests, I see that all time, but never enough to stop the drug. Only about 0.1% of patients get symptomatic hepatitis and it is mostly age-related, and perhaps worse in women. Given the relatively rarity of symptomatic INH hepatitis, I am not surprised it is my first.

How about alcohol use? Ethanol is a known hepatotoxin and it should potentiate the effects of INH. Right?

The data is relatively sparse, although *Clinical Infectious Diseases* says, "It is well established that alcohol use while taking isoniazid increases the incidence of hepatitis."

Well established. Must mean lots of quality data. Everyone seems to refer to one study:

"In the USPHS surveillance study (63), alcohol consumption appeared to more than double the rate of probable isoniazid hepatitis, with daily consumption increasing the rate more than four times."

which is the only reference in the CDC guidelines for INH/Alcohol related hepatitis.

Another study demonstrated

*"There was **no association** between hepatotoxicity and gender, race/ethnicity, **self-reported alcohol consumption**, or self-reported history of previous liver disease"*

and another

*"Risk factors of hepatotoxicity included old age, female sex and extensive tuberculosis, and **not alcohol consumption**."*

And another

*"Of the various risk factors analyzed, only advanced age, hypoalbuminaemia, **high alcohol intake**, slow acetylator phenotype, and extensive disease were risk factors for the development of hepatotoxicity."*

Although some studies were treatment of active TB, not prophylaxis of latent TB.

The guidelines always make it appear that ANY alcohol is to be avoided, but I can see no reason why a glass of wine with dinner or a beer on a hot day is going to adversely affect my liver. When I converted my PPD as a fellow (source unknown) I called it my year without beer, although I had the odd IPA on the weekend with no ill effect. Of course, such an anecdote is absolutely worthless.

Still, when I talk to patients, I tell them no alcohol, but not with a lot of enthusiasm that I have the data to back the recommendations.

Rationalization

Am J Respir Crit Care Med. 2006 Oct 15;174(8):935-52. An official ATS statement: hepatotoxicity of antituberculosis therapy. http://www.ncbi.nlm.nih.gov/pubmed/17021358

Treatment of Latent Tuberculosis Infection in Patients Aged ≥35 Years Clinical Infectious Diseases Volume 31, Issue 3 Pp. 826-829 http://www.ncbi.nlm.nih.gov/pubmed/11017843

Kopanoff DE, Snider D, Caras G. Isoniazid related hepatitis: a U.S. Public Health Service cooperative surveillance study. Am Rev Respir Dis 1979;117:991–1001.

Chest. 2005 Jul;128(1):116-23. Isoniazid hepatotoxicity associated with treatment of latent tuberculosis infection: a 7-year evaluation from a public health tuberculosis clinic. http://www.ncbi.nlm.nih.gov/pubmed/16002924

Tubercle and Lung Disease Volume 77, Issue 4, August 1996, Pages 335-340 Liver injury during antituberculosis treatment: An 11-year study

Thorax 1996;51:132-136 doi:10.1136/thx.51.2.132 Risk factors for hepatotoxicity from antituberculosis drugs: a case-control study. http://thorax.bmj.com/content/51/2/132.abstract

---

POLL RESULTS

When I convert my PPD

- INH and no alcohol for me. 15%
- INH and drink responsibly. 30%
- No INH so I can continue to drink. 18%
- I'm usually to drunk to remember my meds. 15%
- INH doesn't interact with meth, so I have nothing to worry about. 9%
- Other Answers 12%
    1. rifampin x 4 months

ECHO RANT echo rant

ANYONE who participates in my growing multimedia empire knows how much I love Infectious Diseases. It is endlessly fun and endlessly interesting. However I note that as I get older I become more and more crotchety. There are things about the modern practice of medicine that Drive. Me. Nuts.

One is that the judicious use of diagnostic and therapeutic modalities has apparently disappeared. When the patient gets admitted to the hospital, because of the cost of being hospitalized, every conceivable test is ordered. Long gone are the days when one would do a careful history and physical, order a few tests, analyze the results, order a few more tests, analyze the results, order a few more tests and so on until a diagnosis was reached. It just costs too damn much to keep people in the hospital to practice judicious medicine.

Sometimes I think we act like diagnostic monkeys throwing our feces at the wall and seeing what sticks.

You may say, "Crislip, you're just a grouchy old dinosaur who can't get with modernity." And you would be right. Still.

For example, echocardiograms (ECHO). The current indication for a echocardiogram appears to be the presence of a heart. Too numerous to count people get ECHOs to "rule out endocarditis" when they have no clinical indications for endocarditis. A recent article in *Clinical Infectious Diseases* noted that guidelines say everybody was *S.aureus* bacteremia should get an ECHO, preferably a transesophageal ECHO. What a waste of resources.

Much of the time you do not need an ECHO to make the diagnosis of endocarditis. A patient has positive blood cultures and embolic events and a murmur, and really, what more do to make a diagnosis of the disease? And given the false negative rates of even transesophageal echocardiograms, in a high-risk patient are you going to not treat them for endocarditis with a negative ECHO? Not me. Too many negatives there.

Take the patient in question. Please. The patient has diabetes, is on dialysis, and has abnormal valves secondary to aging. They are thickened, scarred, and calcified. The patient has a sustained bacteremia, two positive blood cultures over several hours, and the source appears to be his dialysis catheter. The fevers remit after pulling the catheter and the repeat blood cultures are negative.

The patient is at high risk for the development of endocarditis with multiple risk factors for getting a complication of his *S. aureus* bacteremia.

I'll get an ECHO if I think the patient is having a complication, if the fevers persist to look for ring abscess or if the patient has embolic events or if the patient has progressive heart failure. Then I will be asking the question "Is there a process going on will warrant an intervention?" But given the clinical scenario, which is most often the case, I don't need no stinking echo to make a diagnosis of endocarditis, or at least treat as if endocarditis is present. And negative echo is not going to change what I'm going to do.

There was a recent study that did demonstrate that patients at low risk for endocarditis may not necessarily need an echocardiogram. What is low risk? Someone with none of the following:

"prolonged bacteremia, the presence of a permanent intracardiac device (eg, a prosthetic heart valve, pacemaker, or cardioverter-defibrillator), hemodialysis dependency, spinal infection (eg, vertebral osteomyelitis, epidural, subdural or intraspinal empyema, or abscess), and nonvertebral osteomyelitis."

As if such a patient exists.

Of course the patient had a transthoracic ECHO. And of course it's negative. And I have recommended a transesophageal ECHO not to make the diagnosis of endocarditis but because I'm concerned about potential complications, especially with the pacemaker in place. If the pacer is infected it probably needs to come out. But if the echo is negative I still think the patient needs a long course of antibiotics because I can't afford for the patient to not be treated for sustained bacteremia with all those risk factors.

Of course this is the 2010s. Everybody gets an ECHO. And it is often a waste of time and money because it doesn't alter what is done. Every test every time in every patient. That's the motto of modern medicine sometimes. So says the grumpy old dinosaur who can't get with the program.

Rationalization

Clinical Infectious Diseases Volume 53, Issue 1 Pp. 1-9. Use of a Simple Criteria Set for Guiding Echocardiography in Nosocomial Staphylococcus aureus Bacteremia. https://www.ncbi.nlm.nih.gov/pubmed/21653295

POLL RESULTS

Every patient with *S. aureus* bacteremia needs
- a TEE. 2%
- an ID consult. 44%
- insurance. 40%
- a TTE and a TEE. 3%
- oral bactrim followed by an autopsy. 6%
- Other Answers 5%
  1. bacon. Mmmmm, bacon.
  2. clinical evaluation

What Makes Me Guilty

I AM not prone to guilt at work. It is not that I do not make mistakes or have complications. I do and I will err. That is part of medicine. But I don't feel guilty because when I make mistakes it is not for the wrong reasons: laziness or sloth or ignorance. I do feel bad for the patients, but rarely do I feel bad for me. I have a remarkable ability to convince myself I was right no matter the outcome. It makes life so much easier. I plan of a life in politics.

There is one thing that gives me a touch of the guilts. I like to think I practice evidence/science-based medicine. To do that I read a lot. I have collected about 9000 references on my hard drive since I started my Puscast, about a thousand articles a year.

I like to tell residents that the three most worthless/dangerous words in medicine are "In my experience." Experience for deciding upon a therapy is usually worthless; what is the data? Experience for making diagnosis? A horse of a different color. That is the situation where experience can be of value.

Still. Real medicine is not that simple, and often I can't practice medicine that meets my own definition of science/evidence-based medicine, and when I do I feel a touch of the old guilts.

Today is young male who had mild trauma to his leg 5 days ago, then the day of admission he had fevers, a rapidly progressive erythroderma and multi-organ system failure. The diagnosis in the operating room was Group A streptococcal necrotizing fasciitis with mostly septic shock, and probably not toxic shock syndrome (TSS). He has no rash, but he is very hypotensive and was put on multiple medications to support his blood pressure. I have seen the rash of TSS not manifest until the patient's hypotension resolved. In my experience, as it were.

So the treatment is penicillin to kill the bug and clindamycin to mess with toxin production. And how about intravenous immunoglobulin (IVIG)? For TSS, the best studied case, the data is almost but not quite there. But how about for necrotizing fasciitis? Not so much. There is maybe some reason to give IVIG from biologic plausibility. Pooled IVIG should contain antibodies directed against the various toxins and antigens in Group A strep. There are no prospective trials, and one retrospective trial had 1 death in 10 patients with IVIG vrs 25 out of 67 deaths in those who did not receive IVIG. And there is the occasional anecdote. But the plural of anecdote is anecdotes, not data.

A series so small it is just barely beyond anecdote showed:

"We describe 7 patients with severe soft tissue infection caused by GAS, who all were treated with effective antimicrobials and high-dose IVIG. Surgery was either not performed or only limited exploration was carried out. Six of the patients had toxic shock syndrome. All patients survived. Immunostaining of tissue biopsies from 2 of the patients revealed high levels of GAS, superantigen and pro-inflammatory cytokines initially, which were dramatically reduced in a repeat biopsy of the initial operative site collected from 1 of the patients 66 h post-IVIG administration."

So I recommended IVIG. I think it is the right thing to do. But I feel a twinge whenever I make important recommendations without the best of literature to support me. But often it is the job of a subspecialist to make quasi-arbitrary decisions based on inadequate data and biologic plausibility.

And to do it with style and panache.

Rationalization

Can Fam Physician. 2000 July; 46: 1460–1466. Necrotizing fasciitis secondary to group A streptococcus. Morbidity and mortality still high. H. A. Leitch, A. Palepu, and C. M. Fernandes http://www.ncbi. nlm.nih.gov/pmc/articles/PMC2144855/?page=5

Scand J Infect Dis. 2005;37(3):166-72. Successful management of severe group A streptococcal soft tissue infections using an aggressive medical regimen including intravenous polyspecific immunoglobulin together with a conservative surgical approach. http://www.ncbi.nlm. nih.gov/pubmed/15849047?dopt=Abstract

POLL RESULTS
I feel guilty
- when I make the wrong diagnosis. 14%
- when I have a complication. 11%
- when I give antibiotics for a virus. 5%
- for so many reasons I have lost count and stare into the darkness at night, consumed with existential angst. 41%
- we amoral sociopaths do not bother with guilt. 24%
- Other Answers 5%
    1. when a patient asks me what's wrong with him/her, and I don't know the diagnosis

Searching For Something To Write About

IT has been a busy week and, more oddly, a busy August. August has always been quiet for ID; one year I had exactly one consult the whole month. This year I have been getting three or four a day. One would think that I would have a British tonne to write about, but so many have no firm diagnosis.

Two neutropenics (no white cells in the blood) with fevers. No diagnosis, no response to antibiotics, no WBC.

Three staph bacteremias from soft tissue infections, all with risks for endocarditis, none with convincing findings for endocarditis.

A persisting high white blood cell count after a complicated cardiac stenting. I'll be damned if I can find why the WBC is 21,000 cells per microliter. One of those cases that defines a subspecialist: ignorance with style and grace.

A tenosynovitis after a fall in the dirt. The gram stain has wood, dirt, grass and mixed organisms still to be identified.

Two maybe aspiration pneumonias, maybe an HIV.
4 fevers with no etiology discovered and, like fevers are wont to do, they went away on their own. I tried to take the credit.

A pair of S .viridans endocarditis in the elderly. That sounds like two valves are infected. It is two patients each with endocarditis.

One potentially great diagnosis, but if the serology is positive, why mention it now and spoil the effect for later?

That's the list as I head into a call weekend, and none of them have any great pearls. All of interest to the patient who has the disease as they want to be diagnosed and cured, but as blog fodder? Either they are straightforward or unknowable.

The only thing I did on any of the patients was to stop the metronidazole on the two patients with alleged aspiration. Neither had teeth, and if you lack teeth you lack anaerobes.

"In seven edentulous subjects wearing complete dentures the culture of anaerobic microorganisms was negative or yielding less than 100 cfu/ml BAL. Two patients yielded high counts of S. aureus and one high counts of P. aeruginosa. In the 13 subjects with natural teeth left one showed high counts of Veillonella spp. (anaerobic) + P. aeruginosa, one high counts of Veillonella spp. + S. aureus, one high counts of P. aeruginosa + S. aureus and one high counts of E. coli. These four subjects showed poor oral hygiene, periodontal pockets and a BAL microflora consistent with periodontal pathology."

House staff in particular mistake aspiration pneumonia for anaerobic pneumonia. While all anaerobic pneumonias are aspiration, not all aspirations lead to anaerobic pneumonias. It all depends on what is in your mouth when you aspirate. Jello and corn chips are more common in the lung than anaerobes in those who have no teeth. Anaerobes are rare as hen's teeth in the edentulous, and if you find a lung abscess in such a patient, the odds are 40% they have an underlying lung cancer.

What do you know? Two pearls after all. Even when I have nothing to write about, I still have something to write about.

Rationalization

Gerodontology. 2002 Dec;19(2):66-72. Bronchopneumonia and oral health in hospitalized older patients. A pilot study. http://www.ncbi.nlm.nih.gov/pubmed?term=12542215%5Buid%5D

POLL RESULTS

Compared to the rest of medicine

- ID cases always have interesting factoids. 47%
- ID specialist love to hear themselves talk. 16%
- ID is not half as interesting as SOME would have it. 5%
- ID docs can't make a decision as to what the name of the disease is going to be. 3%
- ID makes up random pronunciation of drugs and bugs. 29%

Finding Work at Home

INFECTIONS, and worries about infections, rarely enter my private/real life. I am somewhat sanguine given the ubiquity of bacteria in the world, and outside of extra care with turkeys at Thanksgiving, I do not sweat infections. My family and I have never been troubled by a serious infection, and I insist that my spinal fluid VDRL is a false positive. And who can argue with an ID luetic?

But for Sunday night. 1:30 am and I am awakened from deep sleep by my eldest, yelling from downstairs.

"Dad. There is a bat in the house."

Crap. The last thing I want to do is try to catch a bat in the middle of the night. Bats have rabies and are the only significant reservoir for the virus in Oregon. Your mileage will vary.

"Infected mammals, particularly bats. Almost all terrestrial mammals can be infected in theory, but in practice only one or two species tend to be significant reservoirs in endemic areas. In Oregon, Washington, and Idaho, bats are the only reservoir species, and other animals — notably bat predators such as foxes or cats — are only rarely infected as "spillover" from rabid bat populations. In other parts of the U.S., skunks, raccoons, and foxes are important reservoirs (in addition to bats). In some parts of the world, dogs and other carnivores may be important reservoirs"

To date I am 2/2 for catching bats in the house without incident, but next time I could have a percutaneous injury and require rabies prophylaxis. It is my understanding, from the time Radar O'Reilly got bit by a rabid dog, that the needle is the size of a number 2 pencil and they have to inject the vaccine straight into your abdomen. Not my idea of fun.

I go downstairs and ask where the bat is, and they point to it on the floor. My youngest says he heard a whack, then a thump, and there it was on the floor. I think the poor beast flew into the ceiling fan and is dead, but I can't really tell, so I toss a towel on it, scoop it up and throw it outside to be dealt with in the morning.

I toss the towel in the wash, and hot water bleach it. You know where this is going. Morning comes, I look outside, and no bat. Crap again.

I ever so gingerly pull out the towel and, yep, there is the bat, washed and bleached, in the washing machine. In the light of day, I dispose of it with greater assurance. I put it in the mailbox of the neighbor who has the dog that barks all day. Not really. Joke.

No need for anyone to get prophylaxis, no one had a percutaneous injury, but there was the case several years back of the young girl who died of rabies and a bat was found in the room and there was no injury on the girl. It raises the issue as to whether everyone with a bat in the house should get prophylaxis.

Nope. Bat exposure is common and rabies, while horrific, is rare.

"A similar study conducted in Oregon in 1998 found that 1.4% of 10,844 households surveyed had a bat in the home during the previous year, and in nearly one-quarter of households, the bat had been in the same room while a person slept."

With two wars and a sick economy, even the US does not have there wherewithal to go after every case of potential rabies exposure:

"Results. In the population surveyed, bedroom bat exposure while sleeping and without known physical contact occurred at an annual rate of 0.099%. We estimate that <5% of eligible persons with bedroom exposure receive RPEP as recommended. The incidence

of human rabies due to bedroom bat exposure without recognized contact was 1 case per 2.7 billion person-years. The number needed to treat to prevent a single case of human rabies in that context ranges from 314,000 to 2.7 million persons. A total of 293–2500 health care professionals working full-time for a full year would be required to prevent a single human case of bat rabies due to bedroom exposure without recognized contact. Amounts of Can $228 million to Can $2.0 billion are additionally required for associated material costs."

Besides, a washed and bleached bat is a clean bat.

Rationalization

Clin Infect Dis. 2009 Jun 1;48(11):1493-9. Bats in the bedroom, bats in the belfry: reanalysis of the rationale for rabies postexposure prophylaxis.

http://www.ncbi.nlm.nih.gov/pubmed/19400689

POLL RESULTS

The most frightening thing I have had to dispose of in my house is

- a bat. 16%
- an opossum. 5%
- my in laws. 25%
- an ex spouse. 23%
- Windows Bob. 16%
- Other Answers 16
    1. the raccoon that came in the cat door and pinned me in the kitchen
    2. viper snake
    3. not me but my daughter age 14 had a sparrowhawk in the kitchen

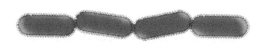

Old Memories, New Cases

THERE are numerous diseases I have heard about, fewer I have seen, and fewer yet I have diagnosed. I am certain there are diseases I have seen yet not recognized. The world of infectious diseases is huge and my opportunities to see everything are limited.

I started down the path of Infectious Diseases when I did ID as a rotation at the end of my third year in medical school. It was one of those epiphanies, like the first gourmet meal or first Bordeaux. I may not remember my first kiss, but I remember my first meal at a great restaurant. That rotation made a huge impact on me, and I remember more from that month than any subsequent month in training. Or maybe it is a form of PTSD and I am exhibiting a touch of the Stockholm Syndrome.

29 years ago Doctor Bryant, my attending at the time—and still an emeritus Professor at the U—discussed a weird case of soft tissue infection. And 29 years later I think I have a case of the same, and I recognized the infection all these years later because of the discussion as a med student. Just do not ask me my kids' birthdays. May 3 and 20, 1993 and 1997. I usually mix and match and eventually get it right.

The patient is in her 40s and three months ago was kicked, hard, just below the knee. Plain films at the time were negative for fracture (although now the MRI shows a fracture across the tibial plateau that is still invisible on plain films) and she developed a bump on her shin that grew into a red, hot, swollen, draining, tender mass. It was incised and drained and treated with a course of cephalexin, but below the debridement site another inflammatory mass developed and it had two new fistula/fistulas/fistuli/fistulae that drained foul-smelling bloody yellow pus. Not found in gourmet restaurants.

Cultures grew MSSA and anaerobes, and a *Peptostreptococcus.* I wonder if this is Fox Den disease, which Dr. Bryant discussed on rounds last century.

What is Fox Den disease? Well, you Latin aficionados will know it as *Pyoderma fistulans sinifica.* It is

"Pyoderma fistulans sinifica (PFS, also referred to as fox den disease because its multiple fistulae and sinuses resemble the structure of a fox den) is a distinct chronic infectious disease in which epithelialized tracts form within the subdermal fatty tissue...Bacterial cultures of affected tissue from these patients yielded a total of 14 facultative and 31 obligate anaerobic species. Treatment consisted of wide en–bloc excision down to the fascia, including all fistulae. Antibiotic therapy temporarily reduced purulent discharge but did not eradicate the infection. Two patients who underwent fistulotomy without wide en–bloc excision developed recurrences."

Seems like it clinically, and cultures in the series grew a variety of strep, anaerobes (*Bacteroides* and *Peptostreptococcus*) and a few had *S. aureus.* I usually say anaerobes and *S. aureus* are not found together in infections, so it was nice to see them together in this disease.

The patient is off to the operating room today, and I will have the pathology report in a few days, perhaps, to confirm the diagnosis. The main feature against the diagnosis is the location: most cases are fatty areas, not the extremities. Still, why let reality get in the way of a good diagnosis?

Rationalization

Clin Infect Dis. 1995 Jul;21(1):162-70. Pyoderma fistulans sinifica (fox den disease): a distinctive soft-tissue infection. http://www.ncbi.nlm.nih.gov/pubmed/7578725

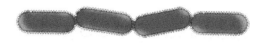

....

Bites

"Here, kitty kitty kitty."

"Nice kitty."

As if.

"Expletive deleted. The expletive deleted cat bit me on the wrist."

Ah pets. Where would ID be without them. Cats' mouths contain a variety of potential pathogens and, like many animals, they lick their butts. I always find it repulsive that people let their pets lick them. If you were to see me scratch my butt, would you shake my hand? I think not.

Second only to dogs, cats are a nice source of infections in humans.

Within 2 days after the ever-so-nice cat bit him on the wrist, he had the rapid progression of red, hot, swollen, painful forearm. He also had shaking chills and a fever to 102, and thence to the ER and admission for a 5-day stay in the hospital.

This pet is going to cost the patient a fair chunk of change.

The patient was begun on unisin, er, I mean Unasyn, and over the next day the erythema more than doubled in extent and they called me.

The same day the blood grew a gram negative rod, and I changed the patient to ceftriaxone in case the organisms was resistant to Unasyn and/or not a *Pasteurella*.

Pasteurella resistance is found more often in the «food producing animals," which are not dogs and cats unless you are really, really hungry. Antibiotics are used in animal feed as a growth promoter, so I am not surprised there is *Pasteurella* resistance in poultry, pigs, cattle and rabbits. If resistant to ampicillin, it is usually killed by unisin.

The patient started to get better after the change in antibiotics, but it was probably true/true and unrelated. It takes a day or three to get therapeutic on antibiotics, and it was probably the usual delay in response. My rule of thumb is once you start antibiotics for cellulitis, it worsens for a day, stabilizes for a day, and then gets better. *Pastuerella* seems to get better a little slower than other bugs.

And, indeed, it was *P. multocida* and it was pan-susceptible. In 409 cats from Ohio,

> *"High antibiotic susceptibility percentages were observed for benzylpenicillin, amoxicillin-clavulanate, cefazolin, and azithromycin (100%, 100%, 98.37% and 94.02%, respectively) in P. multocida isolates."*

Bacteremia is unusual; most of the positive cultures I have seen have been from wounds. Cirrhosis and chemotherapy are the more commonly reported underlying problems. My patient had no co-morbidities. In chickens low levels of Mannan-binding lectin (MBL) are associated with increased infection, and MBL is made by the liver, so that could explain the association with liver disease. I should have checked an MBL level (many have low levels but are usually fine), but the patient was discharged before I wrote this essay. Bummer. I could have really had a great case. The patient did well and was sent home on amoxicillin. I didn't ask what he planned on doing with the cats.

Rationalization

Vet. Res. 32 (2001) 323-339 Antimicrobial resistance in Pasteurella and Mannheimia: epidemiology and genetic basis. Link.

Zoonoses Public Health. 2008 Oct;55(8-10):507-13. Why your housecat's trite little bite could cause you quite a fright: a study of domestic felines on the occurrence and antibiotic susceptibility of Pasteurella multocida. http://www.ncbi.nlm.nih.gov/pubmed/18811910

Comp Immunol Microbiol Infect Dis. 2010 May;33(3):183-95. Epub 2008 Oct 15. Mannan-binding lectin (MBL) in two chicken breeds and the correlation with experimental Pasteurella multocida infection. http://www.ncbi.nlm.nih.gov/pubmed/18922580

A Milestone Passed, A Milestone To Come.

I HAD a milestone today. At McDonald's getting my breakfast, they spontaneously gave me the senior discount. 30 cents off the coffee. To celebrate, I drove the rest of the way to my hospital with the left turn signal on. It's my own fault. I grew out my beard this August, and it is 80% gray. So while I look old, I am a mere 54, young enough that I have another milestone ahead: benign prostatic hypertrophy (BPH).

The patient has a long history of BPH, and comes in with increased urinary frequency, fevers, and rigors. He is admitted, and both the urine and blood grow enterococcus.

Not that unusual, but over the next several days the fevers do not remit and the whit blood cell count remains up. So they call me.

A review of systems is negative. No pain, no focal symptoms. The physical exam is negative, no heart murmur. Repeat blood cultures are negative and the alkaline phosphatase is up.

So has the enterococcus seeded the valve? Seems unlikely with no murmur.

Gallbladder? Again, no pain, and the Alk phos was ok on admit. Pyelonephritis? No pain.

So we went looking, and the ultrasound showed that a prior renal cyst, which had been small and clear, was now bigger, cloudy and septated.

The cyst was tapped and there was pus.

I was not expecting an infected renal cyst; I had never seen one before.

There is a smattering of infected solitary cysts in the literature, maybe 30 or so by one review, although many of the reports come from Japan, where apparently they have an interest in the disease.

Did the bacteria seed the cyst from the bacteria or from retrograde flow from bearing down on the BPH? No idea. While I do not mind the age related coffee discounts at McDonalds, I am in no hurry for BPH.

Rationalization

Arch Esp Urol. 1993 Jun;46(5):419-21. [The infected solitary renal cyst. A case review and review of the literature]. http://www.ncbi.nlm.nih.gov/pubmed/8342979

POLL RESULTS

My most anticipated milestone is

- BPH (benign prostatic hypertrophy). 4%
- Colonoscopy. 16%
- DNR, DNI, DNF, DNL, DNRT (resuscitate, intubate, Foley, lumbar puncture, rectal tube). 8%
- Comfort Care Only. 27%
- Sweet, sweet oblivion. 41%
- Other Answers 4%
    1. Retiring!!
    2. Heaven

In My Experience...

Lots of travel the last two weeks. First back and forth to New York to drop my son off at college, and then a long weekend in the land of Oh yeah sure, you betcha don't cha know for a family wedding. But I am back and ready to go, with no break until the endless borefest of a conference in Boston.

The last month I have seen buckets, well quarts, well a few cups worth of enterococcal bacteremia. All men, of course—enterococcal bacteremia is the price we pay for a growing prostrate, or so I believe it is spelled. And once the bugs are in the blood, infection of heart valves is not far behind. It seems that there has also been an excess of enterococcal bacteremias in patients with pacers, automatic implantable cardioverter-defibrillators (AC-IDs) and artificial valves.

The problem of course is old means decreased kidney funtion and, since enterococcal endocarditis usually means something plus gentamicin, renal toxicity is always a worry.

The patient has two days of positive blood cultures for enterococcus and both a prosthetic mitral valve and an ACD. Echocardiography shows no vegetation, but why would it? He is on coumadin and had only been ill for 48 hours before admit. My unproven hypothesis is that, since vegetations are made of platelet/thrombin and patients on coumadin do not clot, that those on anticoagulation should have smaller vegetations, slower to be seen vegetations and/or no vegetations at all. In support of that concept is that patients on anticoagulation have fewer emboli when they get endocarditis. And, patients with enterococcal prosthetic valve endocarditis have few vegetations, although why is not known.

So the patient is placed on ampicillin and low-dose gentamicin, and in less than a week his creatinine jumps from 0.8 to 3.8, showing kiney damage. I think it is a wee bit too fast to be due to the gentamicin; 6 days is too soon to get enough accumulation of drug to whack the kidneys, but no other cause is found and my assertion that can't be gentamicin is met with a polite sneer from the nephrologist.

So now what? Monotherapy is supposed to be verboten for enterococcal endocarditis; cure requires ampicillin and gentamicin, although one study suggested 3 weeks of gentamicin may be enough, at least in native valve disease. But now? Probably prosthetic valve enterococcal endocarditis and I am chicken to treat with monotherapy.

So, for the second time in my storied, or perhaps bloggied, career, I am going to try ampicillin and ceftriaxone.

The first time I had heard of the combination was in the *Annals* a few years back, and now there is a skosh more in the literature about the combination in the treatment of endocarditis.

Since that reprot there have been a few more cases of success and failure with the combination, which, in the test tube, is synergistic. Probably better than alternative agents.

Two cases is "In my experience" where three becomes "In case after case." So if it works, in my experience...

As an aside, this was written in 2011 and by 2017, ampicillin and ceftriaxone had become the treatment of choice for enterococcal endocarditis.

Rationalization

Olaison L, Schadewitz K; Swedish Society of Infectious Diseases Quality Assurance Study Group for Endocarditis. Enterococcal endocarditis in Sweden, 1995–1999: can shorter therapy with amino-gly-osides be used? Clin Infect Dis. 2002;34:159–166.

European Journal of Clinical Microbiology & Infectious Diseases Volume 24, Number 10, 665-670, DOI: 10.1007/s10096-005-0007-9 Enterococcal prosthetic valve infective endocarditis: report of 45 episodes from the International Collaboration on Endocarditis-merged database

Brief communication: treatment of Enterococcus faecalis endocarditis with ampicillin plus ceftriaxone. Ann Intern Med. 2007 Apr 17;146(8):574-9.

Scand J Infect Dis. 2008;40(11-12):968-72. Success of ampicillin plus ceftriaxone rescue therapy for a relapse of Enterococcus faecalis native-valve endocarditis and in vitro data on double beta-lactam activity.

Trying To Classify an LBB

THE call is to see a patient with a fever and a rash. Again. I hate skin diseases, mostly as I do not have good visual pattern recognition. Histology almost did me in as a medical student as I could never see the three-dimensional structure from looking at the two-dimensional slides. Liver triads? Give me a break. All I saw was red and purple. I probably would not recognize Prince if he were bleeding badly. But I guessed enough right on the practical to pass, and here I am today. You know what the call the person who graduates last in medical school? Doctor.

Rashes often look the same to me. Some have characteristic features, like Erythema nodosum or Ecthyma grangrenosum, which are like bald eagles. Even I can tell what the rash is. But most are a patchy maculopapular erythema, the little brown birds of medicine. They all look alike to me. So rather than try and make the diagnosis on the basis of the rash, I try and make the diagnosis on the basis of the history and disease pattern, and then claim the rash is characteristic of whatever disease I think the patient has.

The patient has fevers and a diffuse patchy maculopapular erythroderma. Conjunctiva are red, but not a suffusion. Palms and soles maybe spared. No help. No real ID history of note except a new sexual partner. What led her to the hospital was a delirium. She was not oriented, although her neck was not stiff and a CT scan of her head was fine.

Screening labs were fine except for a mild leukocytosis and. The lumbar puncture had elevated protein of 240 milligrams per deciliter (less than 45 is normal), normal glucose and 11 white blood cells per microliter (less than 2 is normal).

So what diseases cause a fever, rash, and meningoencephalitis in the Great Pacific Northwest? West Nile. Still waiting for a homegrown case. Acute HIV. No lymphopenia, no sore throat, no adenopathy. Leptospirosis? No water exposure. Enterovirus? It is the season, but it usually causes a meningitis, not an encephalitis. Some weird arbovirus that I can't diagnosis? Maybe. We have no Western Equine Encephalitis, Venezuelan Equine Encephalitis , St. Louis Encephalitis, etc., but as Jamestown Virus showed, odd arboviruses lurk in the US. Syphilis? Maybe. Usually secondary syphilis doesn't cause a change in mental status unless there is a vasculitis. And the palms and soles should be more involved in syphilis.

So we sent off for most of the above, and the CSF syphilis test (rapid plasma reagin or RPR) is positive; the peripheral RPR is highly positive at 1:8. So I am calling it meningovascular syphilis or maybe syphilitic meningitis or maybe secondary syphilis with CNS vasculitis or what? She has features of tertiary disease (CNS), although the rash and fever are clinically more like secondary. Worse than trying to classify little brown bird: this is more of an Archaeopteryx.

The HIV test is positive, so the HIV is probably altering the course of the disease, having it clinically behave like a combination of secondary and tertiary disease. At least I can kill the beast with a course of antibiotics, although duration of therapy in HIV is still unsettled, since HIV patients have a slower serologic response.

Rationalization

N Engl J Med. 1987 Jun 18;316(25):1569-72. Alteration in the natural history of neurosyphilis by concurrent infection with the human immunodeficiency virus. http://www.ncbi.nlm.nih.gov/pubmed?term=3587290

Morbidity and Mortality Weekly Report (MMWR) Human Jamestown Canyon Virus Infection —- Montana, 2009 May 27, 2011 / 60(20);652-655
http://www.cdc.gov/mmwr/preview/mmwrhtml/mm6020a3.htm

Clin Infect Dis. 2009 Nov 15;49(10):1505-11.Factors determining serologic response to treatment in patients with syphilis. http://www. ncbi.nlm.nih.gov/pubmed?term=19842977

....

One Would Think They Would Know Better

You would think they would know better.
The patient has had pneumonia for maybe two months, very slow to respond. It was diagnosed at outside emergent care, where she presented with a mostly non-productive cough, fevers and failure to thrive. To judge from the outside reports, the chest x-ray changes took up about 2/3 of her right lung, but her labs were normal and she was not ill appearing, so they marched through the usual sequential course of Augmentin, macrolide and

quinolone, and despite the antibiotics, she slowly improved.

She came home to Portland to be seen in follow-up by her oncologist, as she has a history of breast cancer, and a CT showed a nodule in the right lung with hilar adenopathy. Both glowed like Chernobyl on PET scan, so she went to biopsy and, rather than cancer, it showed yeast forms/spherules. You may have guessed that the outside emergi-center was in Arizona, where the patient winters.

ID is all about associations. You say tomato, I say *Salmonella*, You say potato, I say botulism. It makes me fun at parties, since all topics have some sort of infectious association. Could be why I spend most nights at home. But if you say Arizona, after an expletive at McCain for inflicting Palin on the country, I will say Coccidiomycosis, which is what this patient had.

You would think in an endemic area they would know to look for cocci, but evidently it is missed in the acute care setting all the time in Arizona and treated with antibiotics.

"A high proportion (81%) of persons with valley fever were prescribed an initial course of antimicrobial drugs. Of these, 12 patients, 3 of whom were diagnosed with valley fever, received 2 courses of these drugs."

I can see that happening in Oregon, but Arizona? Oh well, let those who live in glass houses be the first to get stoned.

The most impressive missed case of Coccidiomycosis I have seen was in an AIDS patient who had spent all of 48 hours in Coccidiomycosis country when he had moved to Portland from the east coast 20 years earlier. It reactivated, disseminated, and killed him. The other was a smoking trucker, traveling back and forth from Portland to LA, who had a chronic pneumonia, atypical cells on bronchoscopy and was thought to have lung cancer and had a pneumonectomy. He had Coccidiomycosis on pathology, not cancer. He was not happy when told of the diagnosis.

Coccidiomycosis in the Northwest is often discovered serendipitously, unless they get an ID consult first: I ask a exposure history of every patient I see. This is the first time the diagnosis was suggested on a PET scan, which can glow with infection. PET scans may have good utility in evaluations of fever of unknown origin, but often will not be paid for unless you are looking for cancer. There is one case of Coccidiomycosis being misidentified as cancer by PET, and will probably not be the last.

Although she is getting better, I treated with fluconazole due to recent chemo and sent off a blood test to see what her chance of disseminated disease is. It was negative.

Rationalization

Emerg Infect Dis. 2006 Jun;12(6):958-62. Coccidioidomycosis as a common cause of community-acquired pneumonia. http://www.ncbi.nlm.nih.gov/pubmed/16707052

Eur J Nucl Med Mol Imaging. 2010 October; 37(10): 1986–1991. FDG-PET/CT in infections: the imaging method of choice? http://www.ncbi.nlm.nih.gov/pmc/articles/PMC2933007/?tool=pubmed

Pulmonary coccidioidomycosis with peritoneal involvement mimicking lung cancer with peritoneal carcinomatosis. Chung CR, Lee YC, Rhee YK, Chung MJ, Hong YK, Kweon EY, Park SJ. Am J Respir Crit Care Med. 2011 http://www.ncbi.nlm.nih.gov/pubmed/21193791

Two Fer

I LOVE *foie gras*. Especially fried. Best liver ever. One trip to France we were in the *foie gras* center of the country and I tried to have a little with every meal. It is good to be at the top of the food chain.

In the States the only liver I see is at work, and usually pus-filled. Could almost put one off liver. Almost. Today I had a set of liver infections.

Both patients were Hispanic. Both had right upper quadrant pain, fevers, leukocytosis and elevated liver function tests. Both had large, septated, complicated liver collections in their livers on CT scan. Both had them drained by interventional radiology.

And that is where the similarities ended.

One had a history of gastrointestinal surgery and biliary

scarring and obstruction, with a chronic biliary stent that had slipped out of place and was no longer draining. The fluid was pus, had mixed bacteria on stains and grew *S. anginosis, Bacteroides,* and *Prevotella.* 2 anaerobes and a streptococcus, pretty typical. *S. anginosis,* as I have mentioned before, is the streptococcus that causes abscess, and is commonly found in liver abscesses. So drainage and a course of antibiotics and I expect cure.

The other had no reason for a liver abscess, being a young—now that I am 54 the upper limit of normal to define young is 49—and otherwise fit. No gastrointestinal reasons, no bacteremia reasons for a liver abscess. And the fluid was brown and bloody. Gram stain shows no white blood cells and no organisms. For some reason radiology had put *Echinococcus* in their note, but it did not look like *Echinococcus* on CT to my eye and *Echinococcus* usually neither causes fevers nor leukocytosis nor a transaminitis. Three nouns following the neither. One too many.

I think it is *Entamoeba histolytica* in the liver, my first this century, and I changed the patient from Uni-Sin (my preferred spelling) to metronidazole and sent off serology (positive). I am not certain as of yet where he picked up the amoeba; he only recently moved to the US and could have been exposed in Mexico or as part of agricultural work.

They say, whoever they is, or are, that things come in threes. I saw a pair of liver abscesses today, so I guess I am owed a third.

Rationalization

Curr Gastroenterol Rep. 2004 Aug;6(4):273-9. Pyogenic and amebic liver abscesses. http://www.ncbi.nlm.nih.gov/pubmed/15245694